#21205 $2.25

BE GLAD YOU'RE NEUROTIC

"Neurotics, of course, are definitely different. Thousands have learned to understand these underlying assets they possess, have harnessed and directed their energy and have achieved superlative success. Unfortunately, many more thousands ... do not yet realize that nowadays help is at hand to overcome neurotic states, to find themselves and to gain the health, success and happiness that is their rightful due." From the "Preface."

Be Glad You're Neurotic

Louis E. Bisch, M.D.

McGraw-Hill Book Company, Inc.
New York Toronto London

SECOND REVISED EDITION

Printed in the United States of America

121314151617 MUMU 765

ISBN 07-005390-1

To

HENRIETTE

My Wife

CONTENTS

Contents

PREFACE

EVERYBODY IS BECOMING PSYCHIATRIC-minded these days. Men and women in all walks of life are realizing that to discover "what makes you tick" is even more important than the basic knowledge acquired in school as to how your other organs function. All of us think, feel and act more or less alike in certain general ways. Each of us, however, also reacts differently, in a highly individualized way, to any given circumstance. It is these *individual differences* that can "make or break" you.

Neurotics, of course, are definitely different. Thousands have learned to understand these underlying assets they possess, have harnessed and directed their energy and have achieved superlative success. Unfortunately, many more thousands still exist who do not yet realize that nowadays help is at hand to overcome neurotic states, to find themselves and to gain the health, success and happiness that is their rightful due.

Feeling frustrated and miserable, the average neurotic cannot possibly imagine how he could *be glad.* That is the history of all neurotics whom I have ever known or treated professionally. They were unaware of the potential abilities they possessed. Once they understood, of course, and found how really simple and easy it was to put these abilities to work, they truly *were glad.*

Preface

This book was first printed ten years ago and immediately became a "best seller." Since then its continued enthusiastic reception by the general reading public, as well as the hundreds of letters received attesting to the personal aid it has given, justifies the hope, expressed in the first edition, that it fills a real need. Psychiatry, however, now marches on at a rapid pace. This revised and enlarged edition has therefore been brought out to assist the neurotic still further and even more effectively in the light of new scientific knowledge since discovered.

A small part of this material was first printed in *Reader's Digest*, *Cosmopolitan*, *Psychology* and *American Mercury* magazines. To these my sincere thanks are due.

LOUIS E. BISCH.

New York, N. Y.

BE
GLAD
YOU'RE
NEUROTIC

Chapter I

I'M A NEUROTIC MYSELF AND DELIGHTED

WHEN I TOLD MY WIFE I INTENDED WRITING this chapter she looked at me in amazement. "Surely you're not serious?" she said.

"Why not?" I retorted. "Why shouldn't I admit being neurotic with as little hesitation as confessing, say, my weakness for tobacco, Angora cats, bronzes or the dancing of the Radio City Rockettes?"

"You're a *doctor*, that's why! Your patients might think—well, being neurotic and then attempting to *cure* neurotics—isn't it like the blind trying to lead the blind?"

I saw her point. In fact, I had anticipated it. And in self-defense I had resolved to say something like: "Don't you see, being a neurotic myself it is easier for me to understand my patients and to help them more?" I had even thought of supporting this contention with an old joke of mine, credited to the eminent Kraepelin, that one cannot be a good alienist without being somewhat alienated oneself.

None of which, of course, I did.

My wife's opposition, nevertheless, served a useful purpose. It emphasized what everybody thinks: that being neurotic is something to hide, something to be ashamed of, something about which one surely never boasts.

But the truth is I'm delighted to be neurotic. I'm delighted because I know what being neurotic means.

That's why I want to reassure all the neurotics who may read this book. I want to allay their doubts and fears, stop their self-accusations, remove their guilt and convictions of inferiority. I want neurotics to realize what they *really* are, not what others would have them believe they are.

Particularly do I want to prove that the neurotic, instead of being handicapped, actually is in possession of an asset. Therefore I say, *be glad you're neurotic!*

"But, my dear doctor," I seem to hear someone protest, "I thought a neurotic state could not be cured?"

"Stuff and nonsense!" is my answer.

Out of the hundreds of neurotic cases I have treated in the past thirty-five years of special practice, there have been mighty few that I considered hopeless. Even these were improvable. What's more, not only have I been able to promise relief, I have been able to say that the sufferings that were blighting their lives, making the future seem like a blind alley ending in black despair, would turn out eventually to be blessings in disguise. Often after only a few short months these same people had a different story to tell. With the hangdog look gone, with the step more elastic, with courage in the voice—not to mention such a trifle as the disappearance of the symptoms—they had to admit that I was right.

So famous a psychologist as Jung has said that all neurotics possess the elements of genius. To be sure, not every neurotic man, woman and child will some day become an Edison, a George Bernard Shaw, a Jane Addams, a Schumann-Heink or a Yehudi Menuhin. Yet it is astonishing how often there have come to light, while under treatment, abilities never before suspected, ambitions but vaguely formulated, sources of happiness never dreamed of. Nor should we overlook the tremendous dynamic force and purpose which all persons invariably discover in themselves once they realize what a neurosis is.

So many hundreds of thousands of neurotics exist the world over that there are not enough bona fide specialists to treat them all. Happily, all need not be treated by intensive psychiatric methods. The majority of neurotic states are mild; sometimes they are scarcely perceptible. The cases that are so severe that hospital care is required constitute a comparatively small minority.

Anyway, the line of demarcation between what is normal, average mentality and what is neurotic cannot always definitely be laid down. There are normals, there are borderline neurotics, there are definite but mild neurotic states and there are severe neurotic disorders. The question is *how* neurotic we are and what we are permitting the neurosis to *do* to us.

In the old days the treatment prescribed for severe cases included giving up one's job and taking a trip abroad. Nowadays the very thing one never does is run away. One always fights in the saddle. Attention to the glandular system—the so-called "endocrine glands" or "glands of internal secretion" —is usually indicated on the organic side, and some thought probing, such as psychoanalysis, on the mental.

For the present I am not considering pronounced neurotic states, where compulsions and obsessions are the rule; fear of closed places, open spaces or heights; dread of contagion and hosts of other ideas that make the lives of some neurotics almost unbearable. What to do about such conditions will be discussed later. Although even the most dramatic forms of neurosis are subject to cure, I am talking now specially to those who are grappling with less severe types. Since the latter outnumber the former something like a hundred to one, I want to reassure them first. Besides, the out-and-out, chronic neurotics need a change of viewpoint as much as do their less harassed brothers and sisters. Even *they* should be glad they're neurotic!

Were the mild neurotic states not so annoying and handicapping, they really wouldn't matter. But, whatever their exact nature, they worry a person just enough to make him uncertain of himself; they bother him just enough to make him unhappy and inefficient at his work; they tantalize him with timidity; they nag him with self-questioning; they leave him self-conscious and oversensitive; they overwhelm him with fatigue; they block the natural expression of his love life. Yes, mild neurotic states can do that and a whole lot more. And they do it to persons of both sexes, at all ages, even to children.

There is hope, however, and plenty of it. What one needs in the mild cases is *understanding.* Understand what it means to be neurotic, remove the ignorance that surrounds it, and presto! the malady disappears.

A lot of the misery in life, if not most of it, is due to ignorance. I once read a story about a group of professors who, in passing through a science laboratory on their way to an adjoining conference room, observed a large metal bowl standing on a table near a window. One of them remarked how warm the part of the bowl turned toward the sun was in comparison with the opposite or darker side. The others likewise noted this striking difference.

After the conference, the professors again walked through

the laboratory and past the same bowl. Lo and behold! the part of the bowl away from the sun was now hot while the part toward the sun was cold.

Heated controversy ensued. How could something away from the sun's rays be hotter than something nearer to them? Nobody suspected the truth that so readily explained this seemingly startling phenomenon. This was simply that while they were in conference a laboratory attendant had turned the bowl around.

If professors can be ignorant of facts, what about the layman's ignorance of the facts concerned with the intricacies—to him the mysteries—of the mind? Actually there is more ignorance to be met with in regard to the neuroses, more misconception as to their causes, development and outcome—consequently more silly fuss—than about any other single disorder.

Small wonder then that accusations are heaped upon neurotics on every hand. In family life a neurotic creates more trouble than an epidemic of smallpox. He is looked upon as a misfit, a nuisance. Friends cross the street when they see him coming. In fact, he has few friends. Nobody understands him. Nobody seems to try to understand him. All the while the poor neurotic is almost beside himself wondering what to think and what to do.

I have a grievance even against certain members of my own profession who, strangely enough, don't seem to grasp the true significance of what it means to be neurotic. For what does the average physician tell the average neurotic who goes to him for scientific help? "Forget it, my boy," says the doctor. "All you need is a little will power, a stiff upper lip. Here, have this prescription filled; take a teaspoonful every four hours. Come back and see me in a month."

That reminds me of a typical letter I received one day from a colleague who usually sends me his neurotic patients. "I am referring Miss So-and-So," he begins, "who will probably telephone for an appointment. There is nothing the matter with this patient, so far as I can make out, except her imagination." Then, after recounting her symptoms—her tortures, really—he concludes: "See what you can do with her."

Well, my good friend, if it *is* only the imagination, isn't that enough?

And why cast aspersions upon the imagination, anyway? Are any of our other faculties more valuable? What delights, what sheer joy, what ambitious zeal imagination can engender! What marvelous discoveries have been brought about because of it! What novels, poems, dramas, paintings, sculptures have been fashioned out of the fabric of imaginative musings! Where would civilization be today if it were not for the imagination? Don't we definitely owe most of the marvels of life to the neurotic imagination?

I know what my medical colleague means. He is intimating that the patient in question is not using her imagination in the right way. He would say that she is employing it in a destructive instead of a constructive manner; a case of misdirected energy.

To be sure, a neurotic state is a mental state, simply because it concerns the mind. That explains why I have seldom made the diagnosis of a neurosis without my patient feeling either frightened, dismayed or offended. For most persons have heard something dreadful about this condition, and fully half of those who develop it suspect that by using the term "neurosis" I am trying to inform them in a polite way that they are insane.

Yet I cannot emphasize too strongly that a neurosis—no matter how severe it may be—is *not* insanity. The types of mind in which the two conditions develop are entirely unlike. As children, the neurotic and the insane start with similar points of view. But so does the genius.

In other words, children having one of these three kinds of mind do not respond to parental training and school education as do average individuals. They don't accept everything that is told them. They question things; they "if" and "but"; they argue with others and with themselves. These types see the world differently from average individuals.

That is as far, however, as the similarity between neurotics, the insane and geniuses goes. And often as early as the teens the characteristics of the kind of mind the later adult will possess make themselves manifest.

The insane type becomes pronouncedly different as the years pass, but the important and essential change lies in the fact that such an individual becomes convinced that he is right, that his view of life is correct, while the world as a whole is all wrong. Insanity is actually the most complete adjustment that exists. It is absolute renunciation of the world of reality. It is a self-sufficient state, and not necessarily an unhappy one.

The neurotic also sees the world differently while young. Instead of feeling self-sufficient he worries about this difference. If the neurotic would recognize this difference and not worry about it, he might himself discover the advantages of a neurosis and be glad. But no! The more neurotic he becomes the more he stews in his own juice. In the end he feels like jumping into the river. All simply because he wants to be like other people.

About the genius? Well, he knows he is different, too, but he surely doesn't worry about it. He projects this difference into a book or a painting or the building of big business. He makes his differences work for him; turns them to profit. He can thumb his nose at the world—and often does. If every neurotic could do that a book like this would not be necessary.

I am claiming you should be glad you're neurotic. All the great thinkers and great doers were glad. Take Alexander the Great, Caesar and Napoleon. Consider Michelangelo, Pascal, Pope, our own Poe, O. Henry and Walt Whitman. And what of Molière, Heine, Stevenson, Lafcadio Hearn, Goldsmith, Fielding? The list could be lengthened almost indefinitely and made to include the outstanding personalities of the present day. Every single one of them was neurotic. Their own contemporaries considered them peculiar, eccentric. Usually the greater they were the more neurotic they were.

Only two classes of neurotics exist: the successful and the unsuccessful. One is glad, the other miserable. When he makes good, the world pins medals on his chest, tells school children how noble he is, even points to his peculiarities as worthy of emulation. When he fails, the world does a tumble backwards and blames his eccentricities for his downfall.

Regarding the full-fledged, pronounced neuroses—no matter of how long standing, no matter what the symptoms may be—when psychiatrists treat these, the first thing they try to make the sufferer realize is that there are thousands of others like himself and that he is in good company. The self-respect of the neurotic must be restored at all costs!

Next it is emphasized that every one of his symptoms, physical as well as mental, has a *cause*. This cause probably is buried in his unconscious mind, which explains why he has not been able to dig it out for himself. The symptom is not the disease, it is merely a *symbol* standing for some maladjustment in the emotional life, of which the patient himself is unaware. Therefore, the symptom is really a *cry for help* on the part of the neurotic's real, true, inner self. And just as a pain in the foot is a cry for help on the part of the foot, so are all neurotic fears, obsessions and whatnot cries for help on the part of the mind.

Why not, then, heed such calls for help? The chapters that follow should be valuable to you whether your neurosis be mild or severe. You'll be astonished how often the trouble started in childhood and because of circumstances over which the sufferer himself had no control. Perhaps it was a trivial matter, but whatever it was, nobody is really to blame. Indeed, it is remarkable how much neurotic trouble can be overcome with comparatively little effort.

I consider myself neurotic although I am not suffering from a pronounced neurosis. Even as a boy I was rather peculiar; I took everything too seriously; I overidealized girls absurdly. To this day I am high-strung and sensitive. Little things annoy me. Often am I assailed with doubt. I tend to worry easily if I do not check myself. Sometimes a sense of anxiety, even of impending danger, handicaps me. I enjoy building air castles. I see life distinctly differently from the average man.

Had I not specialized in psychiatry I am certain I should

eventually have developed a full-fledged and severe neurosis. But I was saved, not by a stranger who took an interest in me, nor by luck. My parents had always wanted me to be a physician and at ten I already pictured myself a doctor and nothing else. The neurotic tendencies which manifested themselves in me directed my attention to mental ills. In those days a neurotic was even more hopelessly misunderstood than he is today. I resolved to adjust myself and make the emotional and mental adjustment of others my specialty.

Were I not neurotic I would not, for example, possess the ambition or the energy to write. Medicine would be quite enough; I'd be satisfied. But seeing life differently from others, I am impelled to try to make them see it as I do. And whereas writing at one time was an escape for surplus energy, it has of late years become a hobby which I cherish and enjoy beyond measure.

That's why I say I'm delighted that I am neurotic. Nor is this an excuse, for I need none. Being neurotic has enriched my life and given a zest to what otherwise might have been routine existence. What I did for myself can be done for you!

The neurotic who succeeds is undoubtedly far happier than the nonneurotic. At least he scales the heights where the view is broad and clear and the air rare, pure and piquant. He may stumble and fall and scrape his shins as he strives to climb. But for all that he breathes more quickly, his blood races faster and the vitality and flow and sparkle of sheer living are in him.

When we're neurotic there is unrest inside us. Yet this unrest is merely the sign that we are gaited for better things; that we have not as yet found ourselves. The neurotic must learn to respect his condition; to understand it. He must cease being ashamed and afraid. Knowledge of what is ailing him is all that is necessary. For knowledge begets power, and power, courage. The rest is easy.

Chapter II

TO BE NORMAL IS NOTHING TO BRAG ABOUT

EXAMINATION OF DRAFTEES IN THE FIRST World War first shocked the country into the realization that the average mental age of the cream of our young manhood was appallingly low. To be exact, the average mental age was 13.08 years, and Selective Service records of the Second World War indicate that we have absolutely no reason to feel that the average has improved significantly in the past twenty-five years. These were men in the prime of life, mind you; and the frankly feeble-minded, the insane or the psychopathic are not included in the figures. "The draft," comments Yerkes,[1] "is approximately a representative group which is presumably, however, a little lower in intelligence than is the country at large."

A *little* lower? So *this* is *normal!*

But let us not be shocked too soon. Perhaps, despite intellectual shortcomings, normal people are a decent lot after all. Let us overlook the fact that over four and a quarter million of them can neither read nor write. Let us inquire how they behave. Let us see what sort of emotional make-up is hitched to their intelligence, such as it is.

At the height of the war against Germany and Japan, despite the fact that transportation was restricted and many race

[1] "Psychological Examining in the United States Army" by Robert M. Yerkes (National Academy of Science, 1921).

tracks were shut down, the betting public, during the season of 1945, wagered many more millions of dollars on horse racing than ever before in the nation's history. Walter Winchell once made a remark over the radio to the effect that wise money was getting out of the stock market, and the next day so many frantic "investors" rushed in to sell out on the strength of his "tip" that the market took a sudden dive. Throughout the war "normal" citizens killed and injured far more people with their automobiles than the enemy was able to do with guns and bullets.

Even during these desperate times, murders, divorce cases, paternity suits and irregular love affairs of movie celebrities won front-page space in competition with news of battles that were changing the course of history. The appetite of the normal reading public for the juiciest details was fully as insatiable as during the *cause célèbre,* the trial of Bruno Hauptmann for the Lindbergh baby kidnaping. Since the motivations of "normal" human conduct do not change (witness the spectacle of women flocking around a glamorous seducer outside the courtroom begging for his autograph), it is inevitable that some day another trial as spectacular as that of Hauptmann will eat up tons of newsprint and spark the same kind of mass hysteria. Let me, then, quote the editorial comment of the *Forum* [1] on the Hauptmann trial:

> It marks the low-water level of decency in America. On Sundays sightseers swarmed through the courtroom. On week days the Sheriff had requests for 5,000 seats. The courtroom was packed with rouged flappers, ex-pugilists, society queens and other curiosity seekers who often created disorder with their talk and laugh-

[1] *The Forum,* March, 1935.

ing and had to be rebuked by the judge. An actress declared the show "good theater." These spectators seemed to forget that this was no theatrical performance but a trial for murder growing out of a dastardly crime. Outside the courtroom the trial was commercialized to the verge of indecency. Replicas of the ladder introduced as evidence were hawked as souvenirs. Restaurants served "Hauptmann Beans," "Jafsie Chops," "Lindbergh Steaks."

If this be not enough, pick up any newspaper any day and observe the antics of the normals for yourself. See how they disport themselves. Without the slightest trouble you can find juicy morsels on infidelity, divorce, crime, graft and sundry other subjects that surely would make a visitor from Mars regret his curiosity.

Do you wonder why I say that *to be normal is nothing to brag about?*

The times are out of joint? I agree. But who knocked them out of joint? Besides, are these the first signs of demoralization in history? Can you name an era—start with the Egyptians or the Mayans, if you like—that essentially was different? Inflation was a desperate problem in ancient Athens. The Romans had food riots and demagogues who reduced the rich to rags in order to "share the wealth." Privation, unemployment, the certainty that civilization is at an end, have recurrently plagued not only our own country but any other you can mention. The crossbow was a weapon so horrible that "another war would end civilization"; next, gunpowder was so frightful as to make wars unthinkable; today we have the atomic bomb. Normal people are always getting themselves into frightful troubles and then advancing to worse ones.

Society disports itself the way it does because of the character of the human beings that make up that society. The intellectual status is a big factor, the emotional bigger still. The great, great majority of the people who make a nation, who make a world, are normal—don't forget that—even if it be a low normal, just about missing moronity or falling upon the bottom levels of adolescence.

A person's IQ or intelligence quotient is obtained by dividing his mental age by his chronological age. It is a rough but useful measurement of how smart people are. An IQ of 100, you possibly think, must be perfect—something to brag about. But what does the figure mean? Simply that the owner has mental endowment equal to the *average* of his group over the entire country. A normal IQ of 100 is little to be proud of, for there are as many people rising above that figure as there are people who fall below it. A vast amount of the nation's work is done by people with IQ's well below 100. The great majority of these people act and are considered to be perfectly normal. To be a high-grade moron is not by any means to be incapable of earning a living in unstressful ways. But what a standard of normality to aim at!

Among those responsible for making this dog of a world wag its tail the way it does there are undoubtedly neurotics to be found. Nevertheless, the neurotic is a *thinker* even if he cannot lay claim to grammar-school graduation. Indeed, the neurotic may never have done well in any school or college because his thinking was different, because he could not be a square peg squeezed into a standardized round hole. Nor does the neurotic *feel* the way others do. Essentially he is neither coarse nor common nor brutal. Unfortunately, and because of an imitative tendency he often possesses, the neurotic may copy the very worst traits of the normal and do everything in his power to behave like them. Such variations of type, however, constitute the proverbial exceptions that prove the rule.

Neurotics are constantly being blamed for being bookworms, for theorizing too much, for impracticality, for Utopian ideas, for wanting to reform the world. They are also accused of being too soft, too sensitive, too conscientious, too sentimental, too irresolute. If the neurotic is concerned with one problem more than any other, it is morality. Continually is he inhibited and restrained. Combinations of such traits, however, do not give rise to brutality, dishonesty, depravity and murder. They form a composite quite distinct, qualitatively speaking, from the concept of normal. The influence of the neurotic is intrinsically refining and elevating.

Be glad you're neurotic, for to be normal is nothing to brag about!

To be normal is, of course, to be average. Average characteristics are obtained by finding the mean of all the characteristics of all the people and calling this typical. Despite the millions of neurotics already existing—and they are increasing by leaps and bounds—the normals still outnumber them preponderatingly. The Century Dictionary defines normal as "conforming with a certain type or standard; regular; natural." Normal and average, psychologically considered, are identical terms of classification. To attempt to differentiate would be nothing short of quibbling, a mere exercise in sophistry.

Don't take my word for the downright mediocre characteristics of the normal and average. Consider this survey by R. L. Duffus.[1] Mr. Average, he says, is:

> A person who is married; has two and three-tenths children; commands an income of about $1,200 a year; owns and drives, on behalf of his family, about five-sixths of a motor vehicle; has eight-fifteenths of a radio set; goes to a motion picture theatre every eight or nine days; smokes two and a half cigarettes a day (or ten cigarettes if he can keep them away from his wife and children); and, if he is over the age of thirteen, has half a membership in some religious denomination. . . . We might find the average man reading a newspaper, for the nation's circulations are large enough to give every family one and a fraction copies every day. But he and his average family would buy a book only once in two years and draw a book from a public library no oftener. He is not a learned man. What average man ever is? Probably, however, he is better informed than any other average man in any country in the world or at any period in history. At least he knows current catch words.

You are correct, Mr. Duffus, but one shudders to think what Mr. Average of days gone by must have been.

Let us note the stress laid upon creature comforts—automobile, radio set, motion pictures, cigarettes. Nothing said about honesty, honor, charity, justice, love, aesthetic sense or being kind to dumb animals. We must credit Mr. Average, however, with carrying "half a membership in some religious denomination." Does this mean that his spiritual urge is strong? Considering the materialism that is rampant it is

[1] "Trailing the Elusive American," by R. L. Duffus, Magazine Section, *New York Times*, Oct. 28, 1934. Mr. Duffus adds: "The term 'average man' has a meaning in common speech even if it will not yield to mathematical analysis. . . . Usage justifies us in speaking of the average American when we really mean the representative or typical American. . . . One feels that the average man actually exists."

laughable to mention the possibility. Nine times out of ten Mr. Average goes to church because of a hangover from childhood, a habit bred of fear and the opinion of the neighbors; the net result little more than "lip service."

As for being better informed than any other average man in any other country, what, I ask, is he informed about? Mighty little beyond the sordid stuff already mentioned that appears in the daily press and is significantly labeled "current events." Precious few books, of course, although "at least, he knows current catch words." Listen to the conversation of the average man, and the average woman for that matter, and observe how elegant and virile his speech really is. Aside from ignorance of, and downright laziness in the use of, his own language, Mr. Average scarcely knows his own job thoroughly, whether he be grocer, salesman or plumber. If he happens to be expert in his work he tries to take advantage of you when you hire him, delivers inferior materials or workmanship not bargained for, loafs on the job, deceives you in so many ways that in the end you are sorry you ever started.

If you think this is exaggeration, watch closely what happens when you send your automobile to the repair shop, place an order with a department store or simply have your radio tubes tested. Ask the average man if he thinks it pays to be honest.

Observe a group of workers in protected occupations—that is, civic employees who are practically guaranteed against dismissal by tenure or civil service laws, municipal employees, surplus government workers who attach themselves to a secure payroll and hang on for dear life. Do such people, in general, impress you as being on their toes, eager to please and serve the public, always trying to give the best they have? Write your own answer. The average man—and he's perfectly normal, mind you—is more than willing, he is desperately eager, to sell out for "security." Any kind of pay check is welcomed, no matter how small, so long as its regularity is guaranteed, whether he continually delivers the goods or not. The average work effort of normal people is so low that a very little extra push easily puts you above it.

The moral life of Mr. Average? The answer is "necking" before marriage; frequently philandering afterward. We read about the doings, say, of the sixteenth and seventeenth centuries in such phenomenally popular novels as *Forever Amber*. We think how licentious they must have been. Is it not true, though, that in the olden days they added at least a bit of finesse? Are normal people of our times so much better? Venereal disease rates, accelerated by the war, have jumped to an alarming degree in practically every city of the country, ranging from 20 to 40 per cent and even higher. "Victory girls" have added to the dictionaries a new term for easy persuasion. Divorce rates among the war-married are zooming; in at least one city, Los Angeles, the rate is rapidly becoming close to one divorce to one marriage! Can the normal people of our time look down their noses upon the roisterers of *Forever Amber?*

Practically nothing has been said so far about Mrs. Average and her children, except the intimation that she might steal her husband's cigarettes.

I wish I could picture the average female of the species as a finer specimen of humanity, but it can't be done. As a rule, she has a keen eye to the main chance, shows practically no interest in her job beyond the pay check, is conceited when pretty and attempts to capitalize it, becomes overbearing and snobbish when a man is in the offing, lords it over her friends when she marries, is gossipy and cattish, prevaricates when cornered, spends her time talking men and clothes, believes all the flattering bosh the opposite sex bestows upon her, often behaves shockingly in public, is definitely "trivialized," scarcely knows how to cook or sew and often brings up her children abominably. As for her knowledge of sex and love, two factors in her life one might expect her to be superior in, the divorce courts tell the story.

Should you meet Mr., Mrs. or Miss Average on the street, you would not be struck by the characteristics of downright mediocrity I have listed. You might talk to one of these for an hour and not find out. That's because all normals wear a mask, a false face, and it's mighty deceptive. They put on this false face when they meet you because they realize how to please, to harmonize with the majority, to conform, to fit in, to make a hit, to "belong." When you consider the social conventions normals conform to so skilfully, you realize their masks are as like as peas in a pod. But can you trust this game of pretense? Recall Eugene O'Neill's first play with masks, *The Great God Brown*.

The neurotic, on the other hand, neither fits in nor can he wear the conventional mask no matter how hard he tries. He is so essentially different from the average, from the concept of normal, that often you actually can pick him out in the street. Forever is he worrying because he is not like everybody else. If only he *knew!* If only he'd discover that he should be *glad* he's neurotic since to be normal is nothing to brag about.

A lad of twelve was brought to a psychiatrist many years ago because he was flunking in school, refused to play baseball and preferred to fiddle. If ever there was a neurotic he was one. Today he is one of the leading violin virtuosos of the world.

A playwright became despondent because he could not place his scripts. "Be satisfied to write popular stuff like the rest," they told him. "Give the public what it wants." But he couldn't do that and attacks of despondency would overwhelm him. Finally he was persuaded to consult a psychiatrist. "Keep on being different," he advised. "Be glad you aren't like the rest, with an eye to the box office. In the end you certainly will be acclaimed." At present he is on the top rung of the artistic ladder with a large bankroll to boot.

A woman who was desperately discouraged consulted a psychiatrist. The urge for a career was strong, but she was married and compelled to support an invalid husband. As if this was not enough, there were children. "Don't give in, don't change, no matter what happens," he warned. "Don't be ashamed that the routine of wifehood and motherhood irks. Be proud you're neurotic. You may endure a lot, but in the end—!"

If I divulged her name—as well as the names of the other two mentioned—you'd recognize it at once. She, too, triumphed, and as one of the most famous and successful women of America.

Just sticking it out, just persisting, just refusing to conform did all that for these and scores of other neurotics I could mention. Incidentally, these particular three didn't even bother to remove their disturbing neurotic traits. They used them as a spur, a whip, to force themselves forward, to boost themselves over the top into fields of clover, where the others —the normal and average lagging behind—may behold them from afar and applaud. These individuals at one time were not glad to be neurotic. But ask them now!

The normal, the average, is surely nothing to brag about. It's little more than ditchdigger stuff. There is no originality to it, no sparkle, no flare. Cling, therefore, to any slightest deviation from the normal you may possess. Goodness knows what you yet may be able to do with it. Remember that you are not going to succeed or be talked about, or even be noticed, because of the ways in which you are like others, but only because of the ways in which you are *different.*

Do everything that is expected of you: Be a model son or daughter; get A's in college; marry to please you grandmother; punch the time clock without fail; own your own home; save for a rainy day; be prompt at meals and don't forget your roughage and vitamins; display civic pride; join the Lions or Rotary; budget your income; carry life insurance; and you may be sure all the relatives will be present at your funeral.

But nobody else will. Why? Because you're a *nobody!* They'll drop you into the ground together with your virtues "unwept, unhonored and unsung," except for the paid obituary notice in your local paper and the printed sermon delivered by your local preacher.

No one yet knows what gangster names will take the place of those of Al Capone, Legs Diamond, Dillinger, Baby Face Nelson, Dutch Schultz and their ilk. But you can be sure that the new crop of desperadoes will be followed breathlessly by the normal reading public in newspaper headlines. Have you ever wondered why the crimes of such gangsters and racketeers are followed so eagerly by people who are normal, respectable citizens? Why should the public at large be interested in such psychopaths? [1] Because deep down we harbor a secret admiration for anybody who is what he is no matter what, even if he is a criminal. Don't forget that it's the *individual differences* that make all famous as well as infamous personalities stand out above the common herd.

One of the supposed advantages of being normal is to profit by experience. Consider the Second World War. Did Germany profit by experience in the First World War? Did Italy? Did the rest of Europe? Look upon the unparalleled desolation and destruction wreaked upon the Continent and you begin to wonder how much nations of normal people really learn by experience. We have often heard that the market crash of 1929 and the subsequent depression were

[1] A psychopath is an individual suffering from emotional inadequacy (not instability), which is present from birth (like mental defect), and is incurable. He is an individual upon whom an ordinary stimulus produces an unusual and extraordinary effect, hence he does not respond to love, sentiment, pity, etc., as do either normals or neurotics. Emotionally he may be as "cold as steel," or may experience feeling in no more definite a manner than does the normal in regard to the earth being round. But the psychopath is not a psychotic although he may develop a psychosis. Nor does he suffer a genuine mental defect in the sense of being feeble-minded. Intellectual development may even be above average with emotional development, comparatively speaking, nil. A large percentage of our criminal population, especially those who commit atrocious murders with planfulness and cunning, are psychopaths. Unfortunately, the courts are woefully behind science in not, as yet, accepting the psychopath diagnosis. They confuse psychopaths with psychotics; if their intellectual development be low, with the feeble-minded; and sometimes they confuse the personality deviations of these individuals even with neurotic states. Separate institutions should be provided for psychopathic cases, the same as for the feeble-minded and for the insane.

caused at least in part by fantastic stock speculation. Barbers would stop in the middle of a haircut to read the ticker. Shoeshine boys would dash out for the latest extra giving market reports. Do you really think they won't do it again when they get money in their fingers? Do you really believe that security regulations, desirable though they be, are going to protect normal people against making fools of themselves? Do you think the war-debt fiascos of the 1930's, when we became Uncle Shylock to the world, can never be repeated because nations of normal people have learned deep lessons from experience?

These are neat examples of what happens in this world of normals. That's the sort of mess these minds that you, as a neurotic, envy, get themselves into.

To be sure, I realize full well that I have placed the emphasis on the good points of the neurotic and on the bad points of the normal. I know, too, that worse neurotics exist as well as better normals. I am not trying to prove, or even suggest, that praiseworthy traits are characteristic of neurotics only, nor that normals are thoroughly bad, through and through. Neurotics exist who can be common, sordid and immoral; normals exist who, living on a higher psychological level (by no means characteristic of the majority), display intelligence, behavior and culture that is inimitable.

Neither of the classes just mentioned, however, is the rule. It has been necessary for me to ride the normals hard because you, as a neurotic, are not likely to appreciate what the average normal really is; what kind of make-up this normal, whom you would imitate, usually possesses.

What I desire particularly to stress is your differences. I want to talk particularly to you as an *individual.*

Your early childhood training and education were designed to fit you in, to make you dovetail with reality as it is, to make you normal. In doing so your individuality was crushed; virile dynamic traits were repressed; your inherent capacities were throttled or else leveled and formalized until you emerged from your childhood a standardized, average and therefore mediocre product. That is, let me hasten to add, if you were normal.

Do you suppose we Americans would be so clever fashioning standardized products (furniture, autos, radios, clothes, shoes, breakfast foods and whatnot) if our minds—the non-neurotic, average, majority minds—were not gaited in that standardized manner to begin with? It is the collective mind that counts and the collective mind is normal.

Are we where we ought to be in the creative arts? Consider our literature, drama, movies, painting, sculpture, music and radio programs. The play *Men against the Sea,* acclaimed as an outstanding artistic work, was pulled off the boards after a few performances to scanty audiences, but *Tobacco Road* ran for six years and will probably be revived to the end of time. Complaints are leveled against mediocre B pictures, but the movie-makers keep on producing them because the box office indisputably proves that the public wants them. Think of the illustrations in the tabloids and the "X marks the spot" pictures verging upon, if not transcending, the gruesome. Observe the bargain-counter conduct of shoppers and the "me first" attitudes of people when something as scarce as nylon stockings goes on sale. Watch how people jostle and elbow during subway rush hours. What has happened to culture and refinement, to decency and proper restraint, to ladies and gentlemen, to chivalry?

What this country needs is not more normals—not even the exceptionally fine ones—but more neurotics; neurotics who are glad of it; neurotics who have the courage to stress their individuality and sensitiveness and make it outstanding and telling.

Mass production, mass education, mass anything is all right so far as it goes, but it scarcely makes the corner. Don't tell me that a chair, shoes, a suit of clothes or a dress fashioned by hand, with the mark of solicitude of the craftsman indubitably stamped upon it, is no better than the millions turned out each year by factory machinery. Don't tell me that modern college systems by which thousands receive degrees at each commencement do not turn out far too many educated incompetents with mental indigestion. Don't tell me that fitting a child to a mass-conditioned curriculum instead of a curriculum to the special requirements of the child, making marks instead of mental and emotional development the goal, won't crush the embryo abilities a developing child may possess and level him down instead of up.

In the last analysis, the responsibility for this normal jumble of men and things can be charged to the schools. After all, what can be expected of parents when their offspring are looked upon as accidents, when they have practically no conception of, and still less preparation for, fatherhood and motherhood and when, if they have brains, they devote them in excessive ways to bridge? Ignorance always is a basic evil. If education generally would only stop looking upon the newer concepts embodied in "progressive education" as a fad, there might be hope for the normals fifty years hence. If teachers would only respect their work, appreciate its importance, take a lively interest in it and consider it something more than a meal ticket!

There is something almost sinister in the fact that the institutions that train teachers are called Normal Schools. Here the word normal is used with a vengeance! We do expect our teachers to be normal in that the training they give our youngsters represents the best current standards of knowledge. Yet, actually, what is the case? It takes at least a generation for the truths developed by leaders in education to percolate down to the training level of teachers. Young teachers are taught by older teachers who, for the most part, impart ideas that were fixed during the days of their own training. For one example, leading grammarians are withdrawing from old ideas of sentence parsing, sterile rules, rigid standards of correctness and incorrectness based upon immutable authority. These leaders recognize that ours is a living, vital language constantly undergoing change, and that "correct" standards of tomorrow are not imposed by teachers from within but by users of the language from without. Yet children are still taught authoritarian notions of speech that are losing validity, and resistance to change—it's normal!—is bitter and intense.

Money, pure and simple, is the god of the average normal. Lesser gods are bluff, show and fake, all members of the same club. *Get the money!* is the slogan. Make good in *that*, never mind how!

If you marry for money and forget love, you're "pretty smart." If you trick your competitor, even ruin him and drive him to suicide, "business is business" is the alibi offered. Everything is justifiable provided you make a profit. There was a time when to be *caught* grafting was the unpardonable sin. Nowadays, not even that matters. What, after all, are a few years in Sing Sing with conditions so pleasant there and the parole board so active? Make money the way normals do and you're O.K. "To get away with it" makes it right. Everybody knows that a good press agent and a clever lawyer will carry you farther than a dozen college degrees.

Yet these normals actually believe they are the superior ones!

In substantiation normals claim the neurotics are queer, possibly a "bit cracked." But these normals take to golf for exercise and recreation, then they play 36 holes and bet on the game. They take a cruise for a much-needed rest, then dance, drink and keep ungodly hours the entire voyage. They wear furs and felt hats in summer and straws in winter. They build hotel roofs to represent an ocean liner and remodel their ships to look like hotels.

Then the normals criticize the neurotics for being too emotional. Yet it's normal forever to be seeking excitement and new thrills, to get worked up reading pornographic literature, to tell smutty jokes, to get soused at parties and stimulate the sex appetite to the point of bursting, to chase after an ambulance or fire engine, to gloat over bankruptcies, to keep up with the Joneses, to become aroused over a rape, an electrocution or a brutal wrestling match, to work until you drop. If this is not overindulgence of the emotions and in absolutely wasteful ways, then this dog of a world of ours accomplishes something when it chases its own tail.

These supposedly well-balanced individuals do not even cooperate when a campaign is launched for their own good, such as to immunize children against diphtheria, to maintain sanitary barber shops, to cut down auto accidents or to preserve the parks.

Lastly, let the car, subway, magazine and newspaper advertisements tell their story. What do they deal with? B.O., dandruff, sick scalp, hair removers, pyorrhea, halitosis, excessive perspiration, itching skin, rashes, ringworms, women's hygiene, menstrual difficulties, sanitary napkins, sprays, douches, mucus in the nose and throat and indigestion. To be sure, it's the direct personal appeal that is sought!

Neurotics can be vulgar and they may make asses of themselves. Particularly in the worship of Bacchus can they go the limit. Nevertheless, it must be maintained that when the neurotic turns to alcohol, takes to drugs or otherwise "out-herods Herod," his exaggeration of behavior is an escape, a faulty adjustment of some kind, which is motivated by neurosis, in such cases a severe one. In other words, the normal misbehaves because the average reaction is like that and it comes natural to him. The neurotic misbehaves because he is sick.

Here the words of Joseph Hergesheimer seem fitting. "Normal people," he says, "are almost invariably without minds or imagination. In the main they are extremely stupid. They are, frequently, widely esteemed and often occupy places of power, grow rich, but they have never produced an elevated written line."

Yes, the normals are distinctly "down-to-the-ground people." When neurotics nose in the dirt they were not born that way; they came to it through illness. The neurotic justifiably can offer many excuses; the normal none.

No, to be normal is nothing to brag about! When I study normals and compare them with neurotics I wonder sometimes whether to be normal is not something to be ashamed about.

I realize full well how heavy the burden of neurosis can be, how utterly devastating when it grips you firmly. But remember that nothing is acquired in this life for nothing. If your possessions are better than your neighbors', you have paid for them. When your superiority concerns your mind and your emotions, you also have paid.

What of it, anyway, if you can rid yourself of disturbing neurotic traits while at the same time keeping the valuable ones?

It can be done!

Chapter III

YOU HATE YOURSELF. NO WONDER!

PERHAPS YOU THINK MY APPRAISAL OF THE normals is somewhat unfair. Have they not, however, got it coming to them? Not so much because they are what I accuse them of being, but because usually they are so obtuse, cocky, inconsiderate, even cruel, when it comes to their appraisal of neurotics.

To what degree the talk and opinion of certain normals are responsible for making you, my reader, self-accusatory about your own particular neurotic state, I am not prepared to say. What I do know is that even if you lived on a desert island, you still would hate yourself.

No wonder! Aside from the criticisms your family, your friends and your associates heap upon you, *you yourself* are your own fiercest accuser.

First of all you find yourself outrageously *self-centered.* It would seem as though the hub of the universe passed directly through the center of your body. Or shall we locate it more definitely by placing the axis in the region of the solar plexus, where the ancients believed the soul resided?

At any rate, you find it exceedingly difficult to interest yourself in your work, in some duty, even in pleasure. Those around you seem to have a plan of life, somehow they manage to get up after the alarm goes off, eat their meals, rush to the office or factory and keep a date in the evening. Not you.

You cannot concentrate, there is no interest in anything, not even sex, and if you can afford it you have discovered that a trip abroad left you as indifferent as before. To you the world would seem to have been made for other people. Despite the hardships you know they undergo, you hear them laughing occasionally and you wonder how it can be done.

You are all *mixed up.*

What you are trying to do is put some order into your thinking, straighten out confused ideas, harmonize conflicting feelings. But you cannot, somehow, get outside yourself, study yourself with a calm and cool perspective. You are like a person living in a glass ball. You see others in their glass balls but you cannot escape from your own prison to study yourself as you do them.

Forever are you *self-conscious* and *oversensitive.*

You respond to what is heard and said in your presence, or to what occurs in your immediate environment at any particular time, as though it were all deliberately meant for you. Sometimes you even blush. While sitting at the dinner table, your niece or nephew giggles, you look up to see whether he is laughing at you. Walking along a busy street you pass a group in conversation and you say to yourself: "I hope they won't notice me." You go to church, the minister preaches about the evils of alcohol and you wonder whether you will ever become a drunkard. You realize that this self-conscious attitude is nonsense. You are convinced oversensitiveness is ridiculous. But it's no use. You seem unable to change.

You find, also, that you are *suggestible.* If someone tells you that you do not look well, you actually feel sick. If an illness is discussed, you wonder whether you have it.

Your *reasoning* and *logic* fail you miserably.

You think this; you resolve that. You make excuses for yourself, then realize it's an alibi and feel ashamed. You find it utterly impossible to extricate yourself from the muddle of ideas that pounds inside your brain. You can't escape your own thoughts. You feel weak, you suffer a sinking sensation at the pit of the stomach, your heart thumps, your legs cave in, the throat is dry and hurts, the tendons in the neck are tight, your head aches, you feel dizzy. In other words, your *emotions* keep you self-centered. You are forever stewing in your own juice.

In the end you become *discouraged* and *disgusted.* You sleep late, smoke too much or drink yourself into forgetfulness. Depression grips you, too; agonizing fits of the blues. "Who is to blame?" you cry. "*I, I, I, I!*" you yell back at yourself.

You may hate yourself to such an extent that you cry. I have seen six-footers with the muscles of an Ajax cry like babies. Everything seemed so hopeless to them. Such a man, an army officer at that, once said to a psychiatrist: "I want the truth, Doctor, the whole truth. I've got it coming to me. But please go easy at first. I can bawl others out with a relish but my own feelings are as sensitive as a boil."

Self-pity, to be sure, may assail the neurotic instead of self-hate. That is when stress is laid upon being misunderstood, when he feels utterly alone, that nobody sympathizes with, or loves him. To feel sorry for oneself is more undermining than being rip-roaring mad at one's own ineptitudes. That's because there is no fight in self-pity. It's a flabby state in which the individual is willing to give up, to allow the world to steamroller him. "Am I so awful, after all?" he asks himself. "I must have a few good traits, like all human beings. In fact, I know I have. But nobody else seems to think so!" Although self-pity is a bad sign it is by no means a hopeless one. Even self-pity victims can be made to agree, after cure, that being neurotic is advantageous.

The opposite of the self-pity neurotic is the *self-sufficient* one.

Such a person, male or female, is mighty touchy about being placed under obligation to anybody. He won't accept gifts, the loan of a ten-spot, a free pass to the theater, a lift in a car or a job, if he hasn't secured it through his own efforts. He, too, lives in a world of his own, in a detached, shut-in fashion that nothing can penetrate, not even love of the opposite sex or the slavery of a devoted mother. Such independent persons, naturally, are not happy. Indeed, their apparent self-sufficiency is merely a pretense set up to hide inner yearnings for dependence. Usually, they don't realize the truth until a psychiatrist proves it to them. Then they, too, are glad. When they finally thaw out they bask in the warmth of human affection like a purring kitten in the sunshine of spring.

Another reason you hate yourself is that you indulge in too much *phantasizing!*

In other words, you daydream, you build air castles, you are full of good intentions, you dwell upon what might have been or what may happen in the future. All this divorces you more and more from reality, from persons, events and things as they are.

You, yourself, sense that.

You tell yourself you should be up and doing, getting a

job, sitting in your employer's office chair instead of looking up at his window from across the street. In the end you hate not only yourself but other men and events as well. You become unduly aroused over an editorial or a news item. Pomp and circumstance, such as that attending an opening night of the Metropolitan Opera with its top hats and mink coats, may move you to write a letter of protest. You fume because the public parks are littered by careless citizens. You get hot under the collar over the slow advance of world fellowship or whatnot. You develop mistrust and envy and you curse everything, whatever it may be.

What you really are doing is behaving like an infant!

Medical psychologists have a name for it. They call it an *infantile fixation.* Although your brain, so far as its intellectual faculties are concerned, has developed apace, your emotions have lagged behind.

A baby, you must have observed, knows no other way of registering protest than to cry. Its cry brings results because somebody comes to its aid. You, too, when you protest, would like that to happen. No one, however, runs to you. The world is too hard-boiled for that. The best it does is give you advice, and mighty poor advice at that. And so you feel utterly helpless, not knowing which way to turn. Being honest enough to realize all this—your intellectual make-up taking good care to point it out—you call yourself names but actually do precious little in the way of self-help.

Doubt and *uncertainty* are the irritations that make you despise yourself, both leading to *vacillation* and *procrastination.*

Seldom do you seem to be able to make up your own mind

"Should I or should I not?" becomes a bugaboo that continually casts its shadow upon your thinking to muddy and to confuse it. Often, as the saying goes, you don't know whether you're coming or going. Irresolution continually stops you in your tracks. You keep stalling. So far as your progress is concerned, you seem to be standing on your own foot.

As a result of these "ifs" and "buts" you find your evaluation of persons and circumstances to be untrustworthy. You place emphasis where it does not belong or, contrariwise, you underemphasize the important.

Exaggeration of trifles follows.

You make an awful fuss over occurrences that really do not matter. You keep pondering over them, first from this angle, then from that. The discourtesy of a bus driver, for example, may influence you for a whole day. Mole hills become mountains. The insignificant assumes enormous proportions. Yet all the while you note your own reactions and you hate yourself.

Conviction of failure likewise haunts you.

You consider the achievements of your friends, of your schoolmates, perhaps of your brothers and sisters. In comparison you feel you are trailing far behind. No matter how excellent your record already is, no matter whether your income is great or small, you persist in thinking that it's no use trying because you are done for.

Another way of looking at your problem is to say that you are too *introverted.* By that is meant a turning of the emotions inward instead of outward.

Emotions, you see, must be expressed, turned loose, sometimes let run wild. They should be projected toward something. Otherwise—and that's you, again—they keep you steaming and boiling; they weaken you; they wear you down to skin and bone.

Introverts, to be sure, are the creative artists of pen, brush or clay, the inventors, the philosophers, the research workers, the people who fashion the new and the startling. We owe almost everything that is cultural and genuinely civilized to the introverts. You, as an introvert, should be glad that you belong to so celestial a company.

On the other hand, too much of anything, no matter how good, is no good. That is your difficulty. Were you, say, 50 per cent introverted and 50 per cent extroverted, you would at least buck the world and fight it. You would not merely protest and seek refuge in tears or anger. You would not hate yourself. You would be glad because you would realize how precious your inner speculations and flights of fancy are because you would have learned that they can be made effective (*extroverted,* turned outward) to the point of bringing you success, wealth and fame.

Again and again, when I suggest to a neurotic that what he needs is scientific introspection, he retorts that introspection is precisely what got him into such a muddle.

Two kinds of introspection exist, however. One is scientific and the other is no introspection at all. "Know Thyself," said Socrates. He didn't mean thinking about your faults, worries and whatnots until the brain aches. That's a kind of running around in circles. What he meant was to break into and through this superficial thinking to the deeper reaches of the mind, where our real assets as well as handicaps lie. Were Socrates living today he might say: "Don't delude yourself with plausible excuses instead of real, fundamental reasons. Call a spade a spade and do it unflinchingly."

A lady of forty-one kept thinking and thinking. Finally she decided to go to the park, where she believed she could think more clearly. Her problem was whether or not to invite a chorus girl to the house for dinner, a person whom she had discovered her only son had been courting for about a year. "Quiet introspection is what I need," she concluded.

The lady did "introspect" until night arrived and a policeman asked her if she was ill. Nor was she any nearer the solution of her problem than she had been during the afternoon. Merely thinking did no good. Nor was her way of thinking introspection.

What did she accomplish by trying to make up her mind whether the girl in question was "good enough" for her son? Her labor was a sheer waste of time. This is understandable when one realizes that all her thinking was *conscious*, therefore shallow thinking, that sidetracked the truth as to why she bore the girl an antagonism.

This mother did not dislike the girl because she was in the chorus, or because she was poor and her son rich, or because she thought the girl a gold digger. She was in a quandary because in her inner self—in her unconscious mind, if you will—there lurked a son complex that selfishly wanted to keep her child for herself alone. Had her unconscious, instinctive desires had their way she would not have allowed her son to go with any girl, irrespective of her social standing. True, honest, penetrating introspection would have discovered this truth about herself. As it happened, a psychiatrist had to do it for her.

Thus you may be puzzled over yourself because you are not thoroughly honest with yourself.

Often, the reason why you are unable to evaluate your own feelings, desires, resistances and so forth is because you never have forced all the facts you know about yourself to the surface and faced them squarely. And often do you suspect that you haven't. So you hate yourself for not pushing the probe deeply enough to let out the evil humors of pretense; of trying to be something that you are not.

In summary, we call this business of not being honest with yourself and bolstering up your wrong thinking and behavior with plausible reasons, *rationalizing.* It's a kind of self-justification. What you thus reason out "listens well" but actually it just "ain't so!"

Then those *secret sex thoughts and practices* that so many thousands, often through sheer ignorance, consider sinful! Nothing contributes more to self-hate than these factors. This is such an important subject that it will be dealt with separately in another chapter.

Lastly, may it not be that you hate yourself because you really *don't want to get well?*

Does such a question sound absurd? Consider, however, that you, yourself, in response to your training and environment, have made certain adjustments, neurotic and upsetting though they be. It has taken years to bring these about. Such adjustments are very private and personal and for that reason alone you hug them close. No matter how bad your neurosis may be, no matter how many symptoms may be harassing you, you realize that it might have been worse.

Remember, too, that when you get rid of your neurosis you

no longer can make excuses for yourself. You will no longer be able to blame inability to work, to love and be loved, to marry, to become effective in some one endeavor, upon your nerves. You will have to get started! Getting started offers so many possible complications, so many new adjustments, so many difficulties, that it frightens you.

In short, no matter how much you are suffering, certain advantages can be discovered in remaining the way you are. One may be that you achieve a certain *importance* thereby, despite the fact that it may be the importance of being singled out for derision. You may feel that you are dramatizing yourself. Such sneaking suspicions on your part contribute in no small measure to the hatred that you bear yourself.

But getting well and getting started anew will not be so difficult as you think. After all, the human organism wants to function normally, the body and mind try naturally and instinctively to be healthy, not sick. Plant ivy on the shady side of a house and it grows around to the sunny side. Remove the obstacles that lie in the path of your stream of mental energy, allow it to follow its natural direction instead of halting it and forcing it to divide itself up into ineffective trickles, and your personality soon becomes a power to be reckoned with. You have everything on your side. Just give nature a chance, that's all!

Let me emphasize, too, that life is a point of view. It is not what *is* that counts but the way we look upon it. As Pirandello in his plays has emphasized, reality exists in the mind.

Whether or not a rainy day gives you the blues depends not upon the mournful aspect of the world outside but upon your interpretation of the scene inside your thought processes. If, for example, you met the "one and only," whom you still love deeply, in the rain, the harder it pours the more will it gladden your heart. What we ourselves contribute to the stimuli that enter our minds from reality is of the utmost importance.

Not only do I claim that you can change your reactions and your emotional responses, I am going to try to prove to you presently that you are not even to blame for being what you think you are. The fact is you could not help being neurotic. It was inevitable.

In the meanwhile stop hating yourself. For you and I are going to do a piece of research—a piece of scientific detective work, if you will—to see how it happened that you developed as you did.

I daresay it will surprise you. Such a discovery alone should make you glad!

Chapter IV

YOUR NEUROTIC DEVELOPMENT WAS INEVITABLE

WHEN YOU WERE BORN YOU WERE USHERED into a world far bigger and more powerful than yourself. You were physically and mentally helpless and you became the victim of your environment, whatever it was.

Chesterton once said that it made such an enormous difference down which chimney you happened to have been dropped. Whether you were born into poverty, into middle-class surroundings, or "with a silver spoon in your mouth" is not so important as it might seem. Many poor parents bring up their children far better than do some of the rich. The crux of the child-training problem is *how much* and *how intelligently* the youngster is *repressed.*

For all children *must* be repressed. They must be fitted into this inexorable and set reality that looms ahead. Children are little animals, adorable little savages. If allowed their own way, if given too much freedom of self-expression, they become unbearable. Society would never tolerate such unrepressed individuals as adults.

Mothers, fathers, teachers, nurses and guardians recognize their duty in this respect. As a rule they not only mean well, they try their best. With the average normal child the job is not so difficult. Such children give their parents comparatively little trouble. They accept what they hear and they do what they are told. Parents usually are very proud of such children because they are "so good." They never develop into neurotics nor do they ever set the world on fire.

The child who is destined to be a neurotic, on the other hand, is not so easily repressed, or he may be easily held in check and still think his own way. Either reaction may cause trouble. Such children rather early in life display an individualism, a decided difference, that makes them stand out from their schoolmates and playmates, even from their own brothers and sisters. They are, essentially, supercharged and hypersensitive.

I do not mean that neurotics-to-be necessarily appear exceptional or outstanding in a superior manner. Actually they may seem dull, shut-in, moody, indifferent and ineffectual. But something is brewing inside their minds, nevertheless, and it is not reached by the well-meaning persons who have them in charge. About all such elders seem to be able to do is scold and punish, sometimes beg, sometimes bribe, sometimes give up in despair.

What they do not realize is that the child who later becomes neurotic is *different*, consequently does not fit in, because he has been born with potentials for development that are greater than, and unlike, the average. Remember he is not neurotic at birth, only supercharged and hypersensitive. His neurotic reactions appear only later.

The surplus energy of the neurotic is emotional in character. That is why such a neurotic child reacts differently to what he is told, to the way he is coerced, than do average children. Being also more highly sensitized because of this excess emotion, to be repressed by the administering of an ordinary reprimand may produce upon him an extraordinary effect. At the same time, since there are more dynamics in the neurotic child, special, personalized and possibly greater repression must be exerted in the attempt to make him fit in.

But the hit-or-miss methods usually adopted do not bring about the desired results. It is not because greater repression was used to train you that the foundation for your neurotic character was laid, but rather because the repression employed was not of the understanding variety it should have been; it was not the special, *personalized* brand of repression which your particular emotional make-up required.

To think of your development in terms of instincts may help also to make you realize that you scarcely could have avoided becoming neurotic.

Our four chief instincts are the *nutrition,* the *self-preservation,* the *reproduction* and the *ego* instincts. Regarding the first two, modern civilization, defective though it be, has arranged matters fairly conveniently. In short, if you have the money you need not worry about obtaining food and shelter as did your primitive ancestors. Your life is safeguarded in many ways other than by traffic lights and the police.

When it comes to the instincts of reproduction and ego, however, civilization has fallen down badly.

Comparatively few normals are able to satisfy their reproductive urges in the conventional and moral manner. In consequence we continually hear of the commission of sex transgressions of various kinds. If this be true of the average how much more should it be true of the neurotic? Such a man or woman, such a child, possesses a reproductive urge that is stronger than normal. What he does is worry about it, feel ashamed of it, repress it. And the more he represses it the greater becomes the counterpressure until, finally, the thwarted sex urge breaks through in the form of symptoms.

The ego instinct of the neurotic likewise is powerful. He wants so much to be well thought of, to amount to something, to "make good" according to the ideal standards his mother and others, who supervised him as a child, set for him.

A strong sex urge and a strong ego urge form an explosive mixture. Psychologically speaking, a *conflict* occurs between sex and ego. The result is a neurotic character if the battle is not too fierce, neurotic symptoms if it is. It is astounding how many neurotic disorders are based primarily upon such a conflict.

Think of yourself also as a creature of desire. Or call yourself a *wishing* animal. If desire, if wishing, were taken out of life nothing but a vegetative existence would be left.

Now then, the neurotic is one whose desires are stronger than average. When he is disappointed, when reality thwarts him, the reaction in the emotional part of him is much greater than occurs in the average, normal individual. Most people live from day to day, in more or less of a casual, happy-go-lucky fashion and the disappointments that befall them—the desires and wishes that do not come true—are taken in their stride with little or no emotional upset. On the other hand, if the person of neurotic nature cannot buy a dress or an automobile, meet a certain man or woman or find a job, this thwarting of desire can overwhelm him with black despair.

But don't blame your mother or father, your teachers, your religious training or the chimney down which you were dropped. No one single person or factor is responsible. Your mother undoubtedly exercised the greatest influence over you. But unless she was a neurotic herself and profited because of it, you can scarcely accuse her. You may be glad, however, that you have learned. At least, your own intelligent guidance of your own possibly neurotic children will go far toward freeing them from symptoms and suffering.

Apropos of this it may be noted that what is generally spoken of as "nervousness" in children has increased markedly. In fact, this subject was a major problem for discussion at a meeting of the International Association of Preventive Pediatry at Geneva. In commenting upon this condition the London *Lancet*, a medical publication, said at the time:

> Conditions of modern civilization have made the "nervous child" unfortunately only too familiar. What has variously been termed nervous disorder, nervous instability, or neurosis, has increased in the last thirty or forty years, particularly in children of school age.

What the *Lancet* might have emphasized is that while such symptoms of neurosis made themselves manifest during school age, they really had been in the making since birth. Both the neurotic disposition and the appearance of a neurosis, as such, are a gradual development. Again would I emphasize that one is not born with a neurosis nor does one inherit it. It comes on slowly and insidiously and becomes more and more manifest and marked as the years pass.

Naturally, going to school, with its new adjustments, its breaking away from the protection of the family, tends to bring a neurosis to a head. Or if it does not definitely appear in the early years of schooling it may at puberty, when glandular changes in both male and female children attendant upon the ability to procreate, in conjunction with the stupid custom of making children work harder in school at this period than ever before and worrying them no end with even more stupid examinations, places unusual stress and strain upon their nervous system.

Two general causes for every full-fledged neurosis can always be made out. One is the *precipitating* cause and the other the *underlying* cause.

Stress at school, an automobile accident, disappointment in a love affair, loss of money, a fright or shock—any one of these (or other seriously disturbing occurrences) may constitute the precipitating cause of a neurosis, the proverbial straw that breaks the camel's back.

Always, however, the root cause or causes can be traced to childhood, to the effect of the environment upon the child and his or her reaction to it. Such underlying causes must be found before the neurotic can be completely cured. Luckily, they always can be.

Remember that what you are today is conditioned by what you have been in the past. Nor is it the dramatic events of your life only that you should consider as causative factors for your neurotic behavior. Little incidents, thoughts, feelings, although appearing trivial now, may have been highly important when they occurred. A boy can be spanked black and blue and yet the punishment may not alter his character a single iota. On the other hand, a tear in his mother's eye may change the course of his entire life.

The child at birth is a helpless mite, dependent for its very life upon those who take care of it. This helplessness is greatest during infancy but actually extends through adolescence. The years in which the mind is most plastic and hence receptive, however, are the first five. That is why neurotic disorders almost invariably start at an early age.

At about age five—when reasoning and the higher intellectual faculties begin to blossom—there occurs a general and automatic repression into the unconscious mind of practically every experience lived up to that time. This is a socializing process. It would not be well if the child could recall experiences relating to birth, nursing, elimination, etc. In other words, there is laid down a kind of blanket of concealment and the past is forgotten. The technical name for this is *infantile amnesia*, the latter word meaning forgetfulness. With this self-repression experiences and feeling-patterns likewise may be carried into the deep unconscious that can form the nucleus for neurotic ideas later on.

Psychiatrists speak of the infant as an *autoerotic* being. The child who will become a neurotic is decidedly so. Autoeroticism is an overvaluation of the body as such. It is a seeking after physical gratification.

Inasmuch as the infant up to approximately age five does not appreciate pure mental gratification, or does so only to a negligible degree, practically all its life is dominated by the way its body feels. The baby does not yet care whence its pleasures are derived. It is, however, decidedly self-seeking and pleasure-seeking. It takes in everything and gives up practically nothing.

In the previous chapter I said that you hate yourself because you are too self-centered, self-sufficient, too introverted in many of your reactions. It would be more scientific to say that you are too autoerotic. That is what I meant when I spoke of an "infantile fixation." You never were able to rid yourself of your autoeroticism completely.

What was it, however, that stopped you? Why was the influence of the infantile period so overwhelming?

Because, first of all, you may have been fussed over too much, loved too much, protected too much or you did not get half as much of such attention as you craved.

Strangely enough, parents can make a child neurotic through oversolicitude as well as through undersolicitude.

Every child must be studied as to his individual differences and needs in this respect. Generally speaking, excessive devotion to an infant and young child, as well as unnecessary handling of its body, thereby rousing to excess the sensuousness it comes by naturally, will sow the seeds of a neurosis. Such a child will keep on craving in later life what nobody will be willing to bestow upon it. In the end, repression will result.

Contrariwise, if a child is yearning for such consideration and fails to obtain it in sufficient amounts to satisfy it at least partially, then it will gradually crawl into its shell, as it were, become shut-in and asocial, and develop a neurosis just the same. Again it will be repression that is to blame.

This brings me to the famous *mother* and *father complexes* one hears so much about. What is meant here is a too strong attachment of either a boy for his mother or a girl for her father.

That such *fixations* can and frequently do interfere with free expression of the love-life later on there can be no question. So is it also undeniable that often they are the foundation upon which a neurotic character is built and this through no fault of the neurotic himself.

It is natural for persons of opposite sexes to have a stronger attraction for each other than for those of the same sex. It is also natural, therefore, that a mother should tend to love her son more than her daughter, and a father the daughter more than the son. Indeed, when the children are grown such affections frequently occur, at the expense of the husband or wife involved. The mother sees in her son characteristics of her husband when he was courting her; when he was her lover. Often without realizing it, she becomes too solicitous over her son, holds him too close, prevents him thereby from wanting to marry. A similar mechanism may occur in regard to father and daughter.

The real danger, however, lies in the fact that mother and father fixations are laid down in early childhood and that the parents do nothing to correct them as the child grows.

You, for instance, could not help loving your mother or father. Nor can you help favoring the parent of the opposite sex, unless such a parent has, for one reason or another, antagonized you. After all, they fed you, educated you, protected you, gave you your start. Nor can you help it if either or both your mother and father deliberately tried to keep you beholden to them as long as possible or failed to make you realize, fairly early in your life, that other decent people besides themselves exist. In fact, being a sensitive child, and one that needed special training in regard to the repression or expression of your emotions, you probably failed to get what, psychologically, you needed.

But it was not your fault. Here, again, the development of your neurotic character was inevitable.

Intensive individual study of every child, and from the earliest days of its life, is, therefore, indicated. Besides, as regards the bestowing or withholding of affection, a middle course is usually best. Never should it be forgotten that the neurotic child is a highly sensitized child. The rules that apply to average children do not necessarily apply to the neurotic.

If you happen to have been an only child or the favorite one of the family then, inevitably too, you soon developed an altogether exaggerated idea of your own importance.

Such children do not get enough of the give-and-take that goes with having brothers and sisters nor do they usually play enough with other children. Being in the company of adults too much they become oldish and worldly wise before their time and many such persons throughout life suffer from mental indigestion.

In what might be termed "the romance of family life" the only or favorite child is the star. But the world outside the immediate family circle is not interested in this play and in consequence the star, when he or she emerges from the shelter of the home theater, finds himself a "flop."

Think of yourself as always having been "tender-minded" in contrast to the majority, who are "tough-minded." Is it not inevitable that a tender person—tender in his emotions, of course—will be bruised by the harsh, stern and often cruel world of reality into which he was thrust?

This is not weakness, nor indeed a defect. Brain has conquered brawn. So also have the finer, more cultural emotional values taken the place of the baser and more materialistic ones. Nowadays we live on a higher psychological plane than heretofore—that is, the neurotics do. Their influence, despite the drag of the average, is nevertheless telling. The world as a whole is not as brutal as the behavior of the Nazis and Japanese might lead one to believe. The better elements did, after all, conquer and punish them. We are gradually climbing the heights, even if the progress is slow.

Some day the neurotics will be in the majority. Then it will not be necessary to prove that being neurotic has its advantages.

Chapter V

IF YOU DIDN'T FEEL GUILTY YOU'D BE AN ANIMAL

GUILT, SHAME, INFERIORITY—THERE'S A TRIumvirate to conjure with! Always are they together, always do they work in unison, always do they exercise the role of the dictator to crush your spirit and make you humble.

Guilt comes first. Guilt is first cousin, if not mother, to the other two. After feeling guilty, you naturally feel ashamed. When you have felt both guilty and ashamed it is logical that you should become convinced that you are inferior.

Recall what I said about the normals, how they behave. And how I urged you to be glad you were not like them, but neurotic instead. I also said you had paid a worth-while price for being different. That price, looking upon it in summary fashion, is guilt!

Average, normal individuals do not feel guilty. At least, their guilt sense is so slight, compared to yours, as to be negligible. If a normal drives a competitor into bankruptcy and his wife and children are forced to go to work to keep the wolf from the door, do you suppose said astute businessman will lose any sleep over it? If he does it probably will be because he was out late celebrating. But let a neurotic businessman commit a similar deed and it will worry him sick.

If this be an exaggeration it is but the exaggeration of the truth. The normals are a tough-hided species. Your skin, on the other hand, is too thin, too delicate, too readily bruised. That is why you never have got where you wanted to go. Your goal still seems so far, far away. You never got there because every time you tried, every time you made up your mind to be like the others, to run roughshod over principles—fairness, honesty and a sense of humanity—it hurt and you got hurt.

Nor did you develop like that only after you reached maturity. You were always like that even if you did not realize it. You were that way as a child. You never have been any different. And it all started in *guilt*.

As already explained, the type of repression that was used in your upbringing was not, as it should have been, different in kind and quantity from that used upon the average. That was not your fault. Nevertheless, you were the victim. You were the victim because you were made to feel more guilty than was necessary or desirable. You became guilt-conscious. After the passage of years, your unconscious mind was *filled* with guilt.

It seems a pity that we should be raised on so many lies. Distortions of the truth, often to camouflage lack of knowledge on a given subject, is the easy way out in child training; at the same time it is the most pernicious single factor for undermining sterling manhood and womanhood that exists.

Remember how you were lied to about the use of tobacco and alcohol? Remember all the lies you were told, or heard, in regard to masturbation, homosexual contacts and your thoughts about the opposite sex? Recall the maxim that said, "The wages of sin is death," and the one reading: "Early to bed, early to rise, makes a man healthy, wealthy and wise?" Surely it is unnecessary to multiply examples.

You have since corrected whatever erroneous tales you were told. Is that your answer?

My contention is that you may have done so consciously. But are you aware that, since so much unsound data were engraved upon your mind when you were immature and readily influenced, the advantage then taken of you may still be a mighty factor in making you feel guilty?

My language may seem strong but it is necessary in order to combat guilt. There is an expression about one needing a rough ax to split a rough log. Guilt is such a rough log.

Guilt is the forerunner of most of the neurotic symptoms that exist. It is the root cause for oversensitiveness, for self-consciousness, for discouragement and disgust, for self-pity, for doubt, uncertainty and vacillation, for exaggeration of trifles, for convictions of unworthiness and failure, for misgivings and despair, for morbid self-depreciation, shame and inferiority, for depression, for lack of confidence, for fears of all kinds and for all sorts of mental tortures—not to mention physical ones—that would stand comparison with Dante's conception of the inferno.

Unfortunately, "don't" still is the usual cudgel word by which parents coerce their children; punishing them and making them feel ashamed, frequently without their fully understanding why, still are the means usually employed to bring home to the offspring the fact that they have done wrong. This conviction of wrongdoing is, to be sure, often intensified by the intimidation and fear that school and religious teachers instill into the immature and developing mind. It would be impossible, therefore, for anyone wholly to escape guilt feelings.

In addition, there is not an individual living (adult or child) who has not or does not accuse himself or herself of harboring sex thoughts or of having given way to sex practices (alone or in conjunction with others) at some time during his life which either he has been taught or has heard are wrong. Yet the real harm that flows from secret sex acts is entirely mental in that it produces so much unwarranted guilt.[1] Furthermore, despite popular opinion to the contrary, onanism never has led to insanity. Ignorance regarding the truth about sex in all its manifold ramifications is one of the most fruitful causes for people believing the "bunk" that they must, at last, be paying for their supposed sex transgressions with a neurotic disorder or with a definitely deranged or deteriorated mind.

Although the discussion of sex as such is freer than heretofore, it still remains more or less of a taboo subject and the joke with the double meaning continues to be the prevalent social way of letting off repressed sexual steam. A wrong slant on sex and the love life in general is what causes many convictions of guilt, especially in women and children. The scientific truth, of course, never did. Thousands of young girls, when they become aware of the stirrings of the reproductive urge within themselves and note the phantasies that result therefrom, immediately come to the conclusion that they must be foul-minded. Their ideation then is so much at variance with what they were taught as children.

Nor has the postwar revolt of youth with its consequent

[1] For further discussion and a specific example, see Chap. X.

moral looseness corrected the situation. Sooner or later a backward swing of the pendulum toward Victorian conduct will be evidenced. There are marked cycles in expression of moral standards just as there are cycles in the business world. These social swings from strictness to looseness and back again do not fundamentally change the deep, underlying attitudes toward sex that have developed in the individual, however they may modify their outward expression. Sex remains something dirty to most people. It probably always will. Besides, *mirabile dictu* for this day and age, women exist who are puzzled as to how the sex act is performed, what is to be expected from it, or even how a baby is born! And, "believe it or not," the knowledge that most men have on the subject is scarcely more profound.

Shame flows from guilt so quickly that both would seem to arise simultaneously. Individuals do not know that others likewise are upset. They think they must be unique. Hence shame grips them all the harder.

With shame there also arises the impulse to compare oneself with others; to discover, if possible, whether others know what is going on. The ego instinct now makes its appearance to start a conflict with the reproductive urge. The ego (the personality, if you prefer) striving to be acceptable and well thought of by others lines itself up against the physical, animal needs of the body, the purely reproductive strivings as such. Before long the ego gets the upper hand and the guilty and ashamed individual is led to suspect, if not to believe, that others have noticed, that others really do know. That is when the individual becomes a prey to suspicion, avoids social gatherings, blushes, observes himself in the mirror, becomes convinced that his eyes are telltale, develops self-consciousness, palpitation of the heart, digestive disturbances and all sorts of similar upsets. This is the time also when the prevalent complex that I am pleased to call "What would people think?" arises. Guilt and shame have finally joined hands in preparing the man or woman for *inferiority.*

Convictions of inferiority are so prevalent that the term *inferiority complex* has become a byword. They surely are responsible for a tremendous amount of unhappiness and failure.

If a person recognizes consciously that he is inferior and this is based upon facts concerning his inability to make good in a special line of work, upon unpreparedness perhaps, upon lack of alertness or upon one or more similar handicaps, that person in a strict scientific sense cannot be said to be suffering from an inferiority complex. Nor can a person who is physically handicapped, say, with lameness or blindness, be so designated.

Technically, a *complex* is a repressed idea, experience, or both, linked to a disagreeable emotion. Complexes are repressions from the *conscious* into the *unconscious.* Whenever anything occurs during the waking life that upsets us we try to push it out of the way; we try to forget it. By forcing it out of the conscious mind into the unconscious, however, we do not make it vanish. Especially is this true when the disagreeable experience has to do with the thwarting of some instinctive demand, as noted above in the discussion of guilt.

Suppose a girl, well brought up in the conventional sense, falls in love with a married man. Consciousness, conscience, ego—call it what you like—says "No" but her instinctive sex urge says "Yes." Finally ego wins; the girl tries to forget the man that society, her upbringing, her moral and religious codes declare she may not possess. In a few weeks she succeeds in interesting herself in her home, her work, possibly even in other men. In short, the mind has been able to repress the love affair with its painful associations from one part of itself (the conscious) into another part (the unconscious). In the latter, psychiatrists say, a complex is formed—that is, a tangle of thwartings, emotions at cross-purposes and upsetting feeling-patterns that lead, like an ostracized colony, an existence apart.

Will this young lady whom we are considering remain free of dissatisfaction after having succeeded in repressing her primitive demands? Although she no longer thinks (consciously, to be sure) of the married man whom she wanted as a lover, is that the end of him? Quite the contrary is the truth.

After all, what does her sexual apparatus, as such, her organic physical side, care for the customs of the world of reality, for the rule of the greatest good to the greatest number—here, specifically, for the marriage vows of the man she desired? Her unconscious animal self wants to express itself irrespective of conscious taboos. It wants its man, this particular man. The way it finally accomplishes that—the way the complex makes its escape—is in a substitute way, because it cannot do otherwise. Therefore, the girl becomes convinced she is an inferior. She probably would not realize what the specific cause is. Yet inferiority becomes a symptom, a symbol or sign of her defeat, actually the defeat of her deepest and most fundamental desires.

I have personally known scores of cases like that. Similar sex repressions for social reasons may not always lead to inferiority. They may lead merely to a state of unrest, dissatisfaction and general nervousness. On the other hand, inferiority may result from repressions that are not sexual. Repeated thwartings of ambition in nonsexual spheres as in business, a domineering father, mother or teacher—similar repressions of personality development usually engendered during childhood or adolescence—may definitely give rise to convictions of inferiority.[1]

Referring to those who think they are suffering from an inferiority complex which is due to handicaps that are entirely conscious, it may be added that *exaggeration* and *faulty evaluation* of the difficulty complained of is usually a basic cause. Often all that is necessary in such cases is to aid the individual to get an unbiased perspective on himself and to change his mode of work or living. Indeed, he can actually do all this for himself.

A girl who was lame became so morose because she could not dance that she considered taking her own life. Luckily she sought medical aid in time. The lameness could not be cured but her mental viewpoint, her *conscious inferiority*, could.

Rhythm and melody were what this unfortunate girl's emotions craved. And it was an outlet for this that her

[1] The mechanism by which our unfulfilled desires transmute themselves into symptoms, as well as into errors that we commit almost daily, is discussed more fully in Chap. VIII, "Your Errors Have a Meaning" and in Chap. IX, "Your Compulsions Are Calls for Help." Further similar discussions will be found in Chap. X, "Are You Getting the Most Out of Your Insomnia and Dreams?"

psychiatrist at once sought. He realized that if she could express herself musically, especially if she could be made proficient in it, a substitute would be found for her inability to dance. So it proved to be.

When I met her she played the piano, but only fairly well. I got her to put her whole heart and soul into it. With a proficient instructor and six hours of practice each day, she not only developed into a piano teacher herself but eventually she became a concert performer. What did dancing matter when she could express herself musically in another gratifying way? In this new life she could not possibly feel inferior. She had got a new slant on herself. She quickly became an adjusted and contented woman.

Another case of conscious inferiority was that of a sailor who had once been a lawyer. After practicing law for five years his brother was convicted of forgery and sent to state's prison. This so weighed on the brother's mind that he fled from everything and hid himself in the service of the merchant marine. His brother's criminal act had disgraced him, he felt. It had overwhelmed him with personal inferiority.

Here was another example of emotional exaggeration, only in a somewhat different way. The lame girl had allowed a real handicap to haunt her beyond all reasonable limits. The lawyer went a step further and manufactured a handicap for himself out of whole cloth.

"Did you in any way, directly or indirectly, aid your brother in the forgery?" he was asked.

"No," he replied. "I didn't know a thing about it until he was arrested."

"Then why did you run away? By no stretch of the imagination could you have been held accountable."

"I know that. Still I could not get it out of my head what people would think of me, knowing I was related. I was afraid it might hurt me professionally. People might not trust me."

"You did not wait to find out, however?"

"You are right there, doctor," he replied. "I quit at once."

"In other words, you became more scared of yourself than of your brother's crime?"

After a pause he said, "I never thought of it in that light before. Maybe if I had stuck it out nothing would have happened."

"Go back to your law work," I advised. "Take this inferiority feeling by the throat and throttle it. And just to prove to yourself how defiant you can be and what a good scrapper you really are, devote most of your attention to that very branch of the law that deals with criminality. Specialize in criminal law!"

He did and he won! The inferiority fled helter-skelter!

Still another example concerns a man who was forced to quit school to go to work and help at home. He had reached the graduation class but had not been able to complete that last term. This worried him for years afterward. He never could completely rid himself of inferiority because he thought he lacked the proper education to develop himself fully. And this despite the fact that when I met him he was holding down an executive job at fifteen thousand a year!

Yet the adjustment was so readily made. A private tutor not only taught him the subjects he had missed in the graduation class but high-school and college subjects as well. In this manner the business executive made up for lost time. After a few months of coaching and reading at night he found he could discuss intelligently such subjects as history, literature and politics in any company, without fear of making a fool of himself, without feeling inferior.

Exaggeration of *emotional reaction* must first of all be removed in solving conscious inferiority problems. One asks the sufferer to make out a list of his abilities—the things he is capable of doing—and weigh them against his conscious handicap. Then these assets are emphasized. They are talked about and thought about. The element of timidity is, in this way, replaced by self-confidence. This counteracts the handicap and opens up new interests. That is about all that is necessary.

In the other class of inferiority convictions, the *unconscious* type, the inferiority is frequently disguised. These are the deeper and more pronounced types. They are the kinds that do the greatest damage. Sometimes, if undiscovered, they completely wreck people's lives.

Those who suffer from unconscious inferiority do not know that the inferiority exists. They are made to think and feel and act in strange and peculiar ways by emotional mechanisms of which they are absolutely unconscious. They are totally ignorant of what is going on inside themselves. The inferiority tricks them. They are like helpless puppets in a marionette show, pulled by unseen strings.

Although I have already cited a case of unconscious inferiority in relation to what a complex really is, it may be well to emphasize the symbolic character of some complexes by illustrating what has just been written. In this instance it was stammering that constituted the disguise, although the patient had believed that the stammering had caused the inferiority. The possibility of a neurotic state, as the causative factor, had never been considered.

This young man had practiced speech exercises for over a year. His parents had spent hundreds of dollars for all sorts of "cures." Nothing had worked. It was simply impossible for him to learn how to place his tongue and breathe properly, so essential in these courses of speech training.

Why? Because attention had been drawn to the wrong thing. The cart had been placed before the horse.

Here it was necessary to draw attention to his emotional make-up, which was causing the speech trouble—in brief, his complexes. If these could be corrected, both the speech trouble and the inferiority would take care of themselves.

I soon learned that this lad was overconscientious. He had been too eager to succeed in his studies while at school. He was too scared of failure. He had exaggerated what he considered his obligations to his books. He had given up his chances for a good education and taken a job as a machine operative in a factory.

When I found that he had a special liking for figures I got him to go to night school and take up bookkeeping. In the bookkeeping class, and in contrast to his former high-school course, all the men were as serious as he. Nor did the boy have to worry about athletics or joining a fraternity. Bookkeeping didn't confuse his purposes and jumble his thoughts. There were no jumbled thoughts to jumble his words. Furthermore, his unconscious mind no longer needed to produce a speech defect in order that he might be able to excuse himself for not succeeding in school.

In two months the stammering disappeared without speech training. A guilt complex in the unconscious that had metamorphosed itself into overconscientiousness on the conscious level, as well as into resistance against following conventional standards, was responsible.

Unconscious inferiority can certainly play havoc with an individual's efficiency and peace of mind. But the best of it is that it can be discovered and conquered. Find the complex or complexes responsible; make it conscious. The inferiority vanishes as if by magic!

It is noteworthy that inferiority complexes (conscious or unconscious) frequently produce in the individual a form of behavior that is the direct opposite of inferiority. One speaks of these changes as *defense mechanisms.* They are a kind of pose that is used to hide what the individual deep down thinks and feels but wishes to keep hidden. Such defenses always carry some sort of spurious superiority.

Thus it may be noted that many men with weak chins adorn them with whiskers; persons of short stature strut and talk loudly while the unusually tall stoop and modulate their speech so as not to attract attention.

Other types of defense reactions caused by other types of complexes are everywhere in evidence. Spinsters often reveal their defense when they say that "no man can be trusted around the corner." Total abstainers may be keeping away from alcohol as a defense set up against a conscious or unconscious, but inordinate, craving for liquor. Even unusual bravery may be a defense for cowardice, hard-heartedness for kind-heartedness, a gruff manner for pronounced amiability.

Let it be emphasized that any urge that is strong—and the urges of the neurotic *are* strong—tries to assert as well as gratify itself. If it is unable to accomplish this directly and undisguisedly in reality via the route of conscious and deliberate thinking and action, the repression first forms an unconscious complex, then it takes a roundabout course and appears in substitute, symbolic form, in thinking, feeling and behavior that puzzle us, as well as in symptoms and in dreams. Guilt, with resultant shame, is, however, the root cause of most inferiority.

It will doubtless be clear to you now that the lower down the animal scale one goes the less guilt sense there is, while the higher you go the more of it is apparent. A dog can be made to feel guilty, probably not a cat, and certainly not a chicken, or a species still more rudimentary in brain structure. The more civilized you are, the more refined and cultural your early training has been, the more have your obligations to, and the rights of, your fellow men been emphasized.

It may be said, therefore, that one's guilt potentials are in direct proportion to one's social development. The farther away from the animal you are the guiltier you are likely to feel. And since the neurotic is such a highly sensitized being, anyway, he feels guilty more often and more easily than do the nonneurotics. Indeed, he often develops guilt, even shame and inferiority, quite without logical justification.

In the first chapter I stated that all the great thinkers and doers of the past were glad to be neurotic. It is a fair question to ask if they also suffered from guilt and its end result, inferiority. Undoubtedly they did. But they, you see, not only turned the products of their highly sensitized natures into constructive achievements, they frequently went so far as to *overcompensate* for their apparent differences. If this were not so, surely men like Caesar, Napoleon, and other outstanding warlike conquerors could not have pushed through so ruthlessly to gain their objectives. What they and other great neurotics did was to turn their handicaps into assets. To this fascinating, as well as highly profitable, mechanism of the mind a whole chapter will be devoted later on.

Yes, be glad you're neurotic. It is hard to realize that guilt and shame can be overcome and inferiority turned to superiority. Yet it is a fact. Any devastating neurotic symptom can be turned into victory.

If you had not started your adult existence with one or more neurotic handicaps—although they are erroneously so considered—you might have accomplished much; but you will accomplish ever so much more when you remove the guilt that has been holding you back and the force released by its removal will catapult you over the top and far beyond.

In short, you have never as yet had a fair chance to reveal what really is *inside* of you, what really *you can do!*

Chapter VI

YOUR SELF-CONSCIOUSNESS HIDES YOUR SUPERIORITY

WHAT I HAVE JUST WRITTEN AS A CONCLUSION to the previous chapter can be proved in no better way than by studying the unconscious mechanisms responsible for self-consciousness.

That the self-conscious person feels inferior, timid and even, at times, afraid goes without saying. Yet the truth of the matter is that deep down inside of him he is anything but cowardly. Actually, he is laboring under a feeling of *repressed superiority.*

To be sure, you were not born neurotic nor were you born with self-consciousness, the latter being a symptom of neurosis. Neither were you born exactly like other average, normal children. For some reason or other—nobody knows why—you were at birth a *supercharged* and *hypersensitive* child.

As you grew older you did not, for example, react like other children to similar training and to the influences that arose from your environment. You may have been seclusive and shut-in and did not mix well with your playmates. Your feelings were easily hurt and maybe you cried a great deal. Friends commented upon the fact that you did not talk much, that you seemed moody and depressed. You often had a wondering and confused look in your eyes as though something were troubling your little head. You craved affection and would run to your mother when alarmed. You did not like a fight; in fact, you probably ran away when one threatened.

During the early school years you did not join any of the social or club activities. When school was out, instead of playing around with the others, you ran home. You may have studied hard and tried to excel so as to assure yourself that you amounted to something anyway. You may even have been called a *good* boy or girl. You found it easier to do what you were told than to stand your ground.

During your adolescence the story was about the same. Indeed, your shyness probably mounted. You shunned competitive sports; you avoided parties and dances; you became more and more introverted. Especially, when in the company of the opposite sex you froze up like an icicle. The mere thought of meeting such a new acquaintance gave you palpitation of the heart and threw you into a panic.

To this very day, irrespective of your age, this self-conscious bugaboo is still getting you down. The general pattern of your reactions in meeting people, asserting yourself and forging ahead may be almost identical with what it was years ago, or it may have changed and you have added even more distressing symptoms. Whether or no, shyness surely devitalizes you and interferes with your general effectiveness and happiness as no other single neurotic symptom can.

Then where does this idea of superiority enter the picture, you may ask? How can one be self-conscious and actually superior at one and the same time?

People in all walks of life can be called upon for illustration. Among nobility, King Louis XIV of France is known to have been so timid and shy he was embarrassed in speaking to persons he'd known for years. Yet this was the man who said, *"L'état c'est moi,"* or words to that effect. Napoleon's second wife, Marie Louise, was so afflicted with feelings of inferiority that her awkwardness was painfully noticed at court, while Queen Mary, whose very stature and position indicate dignity and poise, often, as a child, burst into tears because she was so shy.

Even performers prominent in the public eye can be self-conscious! Paderewski, after fifty years of concert work, was still bothered with stage fright, as are Tallulah Bankhead, Raymond Massey, Alfred Lunt and scores of other celebrities.

Albert Edward Wiggam, who has given over five thousand lectures, and is undoubtedly one of the country's masters of the lecturing art, as well as a writer and scientist of renown, was overwhelmingly shy and self-conscious in his younger days. Lawrence Tibbett was plagued by inferiority when a youth because his mother ran a boardinghouse and he owned only one suit and lacked the money to buy sodas for his girl. The late Cardinal Hayes was a painfully shy, retiring lad who reddened with embarrassment when called upon to speak before class. Michelangelo shunned people because of a facial disfigurement. Incongruous, you might say, to learn that even such persons as T. E. Lawrence (Lawrence of Arabia), the playwright, Channing Pollock, William L. Stidger, pulpit and radio orator, and a host of others suffered the agonies of self-consciousness when young. Even George Bernard Shaw would sometimes walk up and down before the house of a friend before mustering enough courage to ring the doorbell.

Superior people, these—all of them! What they did was manage, somehow, to break through and thus overcome their self-conscious handicaps. By so doing they permitted their inherent superiorities to come to the fore.

I mentioned in the beginning that you were born supercharged and hypersensitive. That is what you are at the present time. That kind of emotional make-up is what the famous ones, listed above, possess. You, like them, must learn not only to recognize your true worth but also to have the courage to present it to the world. Thousands of others have done it and many of these have achieved success in some unusual way. What they have done *you can do.*

What would you rather be like, an ordinary low-powered radio or a superheterodyne model? Nevertheless, the finer instrument must be tuned correctly in order to obtain the best results. Otherwise it picks up the stations you don't want or produces discord. You are like that. You not only have a lot of power, dynamic force, within you, you also react in a highly sensitized way to other people—to what they say and do—and to your environment.

This "individual difference" that is characteristic of you—this supercharged and hypersensitive nature that is yours and is unlike that of the average, normal person—is therefore a blessing in disguise. But how, you will want to know, can you make this supposed blessing a working reality?

Consider your *ego.* By ego I mean your personality as a whole, your desire to belong, to be well thought of and accepted, to move along with the parade and, if possible, to lead it. When you are self-conscious, your ego, for the most part, is suffering from lack of expression. It is held back and repressed. It wants to come out like an animal that has buried itself for the winter in the earth and darkness and is eager to be warmed by the sun of spring. Why, however, is *your* ego buried? What has made it run away and hide for protection? That is where your *guilt*[1] comes in.

Let me repeat that average, normal individuals do not respond in the guilty way that you do. Their sense of guilt is negligible as compared to yours. While the normals are tough, your emotional disposition by comparison is delicate and easily bruised. That is why you have been hurt so often, why you have become timid, why you have tried to withdraw from reality and its harshness. That is also why, even as far back as childhood, you have felt more guilty than you should, more than either was necessary or desirable. In short, you became *guilt conscious*. That led directly to self-consciousness.

Whatever the type of guilt pattern that gradually became more and more fixed in your unconscious thinking and feeling, you developed the attitude that if people knew what you really were they would not accept you. This fear of not being accepted or approved, of making a social error or of somehow revealing your true self is the very backbone of every self-conscious person, young or mature. With this fear there rushes into consciousness a score of doubts and uncertainties that makes the very thought of every social or business contact a veritable nightmare.

A young man invites a girl to a ball. This young miss, being self-conscious, immediately develops forebodings. Although the invitation itself has pepped up her ego, all is counteracted by the misgivings that assail her and become increasingly strong as the longed-for yet feared evening approaches.

[1] A review of Chap. V would be advantageous at this point.

"Suppose I meet his friends and begin to stammer as I sometimes do when I am nervous," the poor girl thinks. "Suppose I don't dance as well as he thinks I can. Maybe I won't look as pretty as he thinks I will in evening dress. Will he like me if I wear my hair straight back so that I can show my new earrings? If supper is served, will I make some ghastly blunder?"

So the young woman worries on and on until the tiny bit of self-confidence she mustered when first invited disappears completely and nothing but abject terror takes its place. In the end this self-induced, but nevertheless automatic, torture may well lead the afflicted one to make up some plausible excuse, such as sudden illness, and call the whole thing off.

A man can harass himself in similar fashion. Indeed, I have often felt that when men are self-conscious they suffer even more than women. Being men, they are supposed to be more self-assured. Besides, they are expected to take the initiative in their relationship to women, and that is exactly what the shy individual finds hardest to accomplish.

Such a man may be a returning war hero. He has fought the enemy at point-blank range. Perhaps he has wiped out a machine-gun nest singlehanded and brought back a dozen prisoners. Perhaps he has received a medal for his bravery and wears the Purple Heart. His wife greets him as the ship docks, hugs and kisses him and vows she always knew she had married the most wonderful man in the whole world. So far, so good! No shyness has manifested itself, not even when his wife enthusiastically embraces him before his buddies.

Now, however, comes the ordeal! When the hero's boss and fellow employees stage a special dinner of welcome and he is called upon to make a speech, his throat dries like the Arizona desert, his tongue won't move, his hands and legs shake, perspiration soaks his body as if he were in a Turkish bath, his face flushes crimson and he finds it impossible to utter a single word. Our hero leaves that friendly company convinced that he has made a perfect ass of himself and wishing that a Jap bullet had got him after all.

Nor need it be an unusual circumstance that will throw a self-conscious person completely off balance. A girl possesses an unusual voice, does well with her singing teacher but finds it impossible to perform in public. A boy knows his lesson letter-perfect but forgets every word of it when he is called upon in class. One cannot enter a restaurant or café; another feels uncomfortable in the subway, bus or streetcar, where others can look him over; a man "sweats blood" whenever he is called into the manager's office; either a man or woman may blush when greeted by a member of the opposite sex. Many hold on desperately to jobs they despise or for which they are unfitted because they lack the nerve to try to get another. Bachelors and spinsters often remain unmarried, not because they want to but because they are too shy to try to find a life's partner.

Regarding convictions of guilt, we do not become self-conscious because of misdeeds, actual or fancied, of which we are consciously aware. A misdeed committed deliberately—perhaps a theft, the habit of onanism or other sexual transgression—may bring on pangs of conscience, shame and regret, but it does not produce self-consciousness.

Think back into childhood, therefore, and see how many guilt ideas you can resurrect.

Try to recall how you felt when you began to hear how babies were born and what sex really meant. Did you ever actually behold your parents in the act of cohabitation, or did you suspect this was going on and consequently feel ashamed for them? Were you ever caught practicing masturbation, or were you accused of it? If a woman, did you feel self-conscious when you first menstruated? When did consciousness of sex, or the thought that you were sexually desirable, begin, and did you react unfavorably to it? If you were the only boy in a family of girls, or vice versa, did these associations produce shyness? Did you feel guilty because of sex thoughts you entertained, because you "petted," smoked or used alcohol contrary to your parents' wishes? Did guilt assail you because you found yourself wandering away from church or its teachings? Did you ever cheat in school, lie or steal anything? Have you felt inferior because of race or creed, the background of your family, or because of some physical deformity? Did you grow up convinced that you were weak physically? Did you feel you were not wanted as a child or that you were discriminated against? Was affection denied you as a child? Were you teased a great deal? Were you a poor student?

The above questions should serve as a guide to help you find buried memories charged with guilt. It goes without saying that there are hundreds of other possibilities; also, that any of them would tend to make a person feel inferior and thus undermine his ego.

Yes, you are still unduly influenced by fixations of guilt in childhood, and part of your self-consciousness is nothing more or less than a further seeking of punishment on your part. So you find yourself making unnecessary sacrifices, depriving yourself of pleasure, working too hard or paying for this burdensome debt of guilt in more subtle ways.

Stop punishing yourself, however; be yourself; let *people know what you really are*. Make a list of your assets, of the things of which you feel proud—of your *true superiorities*.

How do I know that you possess such superiorities? Because, being supercharged and hypersensitive—hence neurotic—you are bound to possess such assets in abundance.

Is it not true that you are fundamentally truthful, conscientious, honest and trustworthy? Won't you admit that your intelligence is above par. Maybe you are creative, inventive or artistic as well. Haven't you felt right along that there is something deep within that is crying out to express itself, perhaps in the form of a play, story or novel? Are you not neat and careful about your personal appearance and general habits? Do you not give the impression of being refined rather than vulgar? Do you not possess a strong will of your own and refuse to be pushed around? Are not your standards of morality high? Don't you keep on trying to be liked? Is not your imagination highly developed? Is it not a fact that you are ambitious, feel a high sense of duty and try ever so hard to improve yourself?

These are all assets [1]—ego (personality) builders. But they don't do you much good unless you recognize them, let them loose and give them a fling. When your superiorities are repressed, they make you feel inferior. You feel, as if by instinct, that people do not evaluate your true worth. Recognize these

[1] Contrast such superiorities with what has been said in Chap. II.

superiorities yourself, first. Others will then, and quickly, follow suit.

Your self-consciousness is, in the last analysis, merely a point of view. Once you get the correct angle on yourself and recognize your own true worth, your self-consciousness will cease to be.

Chapter VII

NO, YOU'RE NOT GOING INSANE NOR WILL ANY OF YOUR FEARS COME TRUE

"AM I LOSING MY MIND, DOCTOR?"

That question has been put to me so many times, it seems like a million. People unload their misgivings to a psychiatrist as to no one else. Even the general practitioner knows how common is this haunting dread of insanity. But goodness knows how many millions there are in addition who harbor a sneaking suspicion that they are heading for a mental disorder and either are afraid to consult a medical authority to learn the truth or are ashamed to confess possessing symptoms they feel convinced must be abnormal!

Allow me, however, to be reassuring forthwith. The very fact that you fear you are losing your mind is the best possible proof that you are not.

I have mentioned the factor of ignorance in the first pages of this volume. It is ignorance, pure and simple, that really lies at the bottom of most cases of the insanity fear. The average individual is ignorant of the way his mind works, how it is supposed to work, why it does not always work as he would wish and what, if anything, can be done to make it work again as it should. Nor is this universal factor of ignorance astonishing. Psychology is a neglected subject in the elementary and secondary schools, it is usually an elective in college and even a medical training takes in precious little of it.

Small wonder then that those who note a change in their thinking and feeling jump to the conclusion that if their mind is not functioning right it must be functioning wrong; and if it is wrong it *must* be insanity. Little do they realize that there are scores of normal deviations within the normal; that neurotic states exist that are decidedly more harassing than a full-fledged psychosis; lastly, that the possessor of a psychosis (this is the medical term for insanity, the latter being a legal definition) practically never is aware that his mind is upset.

The individual who develops a psychosis [1] has been heading that way since childhood. A competent psychiatrist would have been able to foretell the inevitable (if the peculiar personality make-up remained untreated) when that individual was eight, ten or twelve. There is nothing mysterious about a psychosis, nor can it nowadays be called baffling,[2] since the majority of cases are cured if caught early enough. Indeed, after a psychosis has fully developed there may still be hope. Over a third of the patients already shut away in asylums leave such institutions cured while half return to their homes definitely improved.

The very essence of a psychosis is the *delusion*. The characteristics of an insane delusion (whether it be in the nature of a persecution idea or any other error of judgment) are: first, that the patient adopts a wholly false premise of some kind; secondly, that his reasoning and consequently his conclusions

[1] For the differences between psychosis, neurosis and genius, consult Chap. I.
[2] For methods used in treating the psychoses, consult Chap. XIX.

are illogical; thirdly, that he tenaciously clings to what he holds to be true no matter how much proof is brought to bear in an attempt to establish the falsity of his far-fetched and altogether absurd ideas. The psychotic is convinced that you are in error; only he understands. If anyone is insane it is you, not he.

Now then, the person who worries about losing his mind presents quite an opposite picture. He knows something is wrong with him. Because of one or more neurotic symptoms from which he is suffering, he is continually obsessed with the thought that he is different from others. But his premises are sound as well as his reasoning and conclusions. The link between himself and the world in general is never lost and he keeps on trying to strengthen it; the psychotic, contrariwise, has broken that link and lives in a mental world altogether distinct, peculiar and apart.

The out-and-out neurotic, of course, also may suffer from ideas that are absurd, ideas that the layman calls "imaginary." But no matter how ridiculous on the surface such neurotic imaginings may seem, the possessor of them, unlike the psychotic, is forever attempting to conquer them and change them so that he may think, feel and act like other people.[1]

A psychotic patient under my care believed all the bones in his body to be broken. Even when stood upon his feet he still held to his delusion. Another claimed that people were "working wireless" on him, and this man, mind you, had formerly been a radio engineer. A third said, "My blood is dried up. That's why I feel so weak." When he was pricked with a

[1] Recall Chap. II.

needle and actually saw his own blood flow, he still stuck to his delusional idea.

Following are the symptoms commonly met with that make people afraid they will lose their minds. One notes at a glance how essentially different they are in content from psychotic delusions. An otherwise perfectly normal person, man or woman, may be troubled by one or more of these and such a person should realize that the manifestation is merely an *individual difference* that, as already mentioned, should be looked upon as a normal deviation within the normal. If several such symptoms exist, especially for several years, the condition would technically be called neurotic. But even a neurosis, no matter how severe, no matter if it presents symptoms other than those mentioned below and the patient is suffering intensely, does not lead to insanity.

Loss of Memory.—For this physical causes exist, or mental or both. The usual physical causes are late hours, insufficient sleep, too little exercise and fresh air, too much alcohol or tobacco, sluggish intestinal elimination. Correct your faults in any of these respects and at once your memory improves.

Regarding mental causes it should be pointed out that the ability to remember depends primarily upon three factors: the recency of the stimulus; the intensity of the stimulus; the repetition of the stimulus. In other words, we are able to remember most readily an experience that occurred only a short while ago, or that was unusual or dramatic, or that occurred several times instead of once. Think of your poor memory in this light and it will explain a lot. It ought to allay your apprehension.

Let it be emphasized, furthermore, that your mind is

strongly self-protective and consequently it tends not to remember what it does not want to remember. If your memory is interfering with your work, analyze your emotional attitude toward your work and try to discover why you have grown antagonistic.

As regards the relationship between failing memory and the psychosis, this occurs only after a psychosis has been existent in a full-fledged way for years, in the terminal stages of deterioration.

Inability to concentrate usually is an accompaniment of unretentive memory. What has already been said about the former applies in every detail to the latter.

Suicidal Impulse.—Suffice it to say that when "things get a bit too thick" and the outlook appears hopeless the thought of ending it all is a perfectly intelligent reaction. So also is it an intelligent reaction to realize one's responsibilities and to convince oneself that events somehow have a way of straightening themselves out. There are few who do not, during the course of a lifetime, think occasionally about self-destruction. Strong guilt feelings often are a motivation. Of course, only the fool gives way. If the impulse persists, as often is the case in a neurotic state, the help of a psychiatrist had better be sought and the compulsion removed. The impulse, however, is not a sign of insanity.

Worry.—We worry because our minds are confused and doubtful, because we are not able to think clearly and to see a way out of something that threatens. For example, you keep on worrying how to pay a note about to fall due until you remember suddenly that you can borrow on your life insurance. The mechanism of all forms of worry is essentially the same. Knowledge dissipates mental confusion and removes uncertainty and worry.

The psychotic cannot be said to worry, because he cannot be said to be confused and doubtful in the sense that I have outlined. He is too sure of his own thinking. Worry can deplete the organic brain system and lead to a nervous breakdown (a severe neurosis). It is often reported that So-and-So became insane because of worry. Investigation of such causes always reveals that worry is a sort of camouflage masking other facts. In short, it is normal to worry. How could an intelligent person be absolutely free from it these days?

Unreality Feelings.—When the environment, including people and things, begins to "feel" unreal (as though objects did not exist or as though they were seen through a mist), you should always ask yourself what it is from which you are trying to escape. Search deeply into your thought storehouse, although this may not be necessary because the reason for "flight" may be known to you. Disappointment in a beloved one, inability to get a job, etc., are common causes. The mind, again in the role of protector, always attempts to blot out an offending factor by making the whole world seem not to exist as it really is.

Feelings of unreality are technically called *escape mechanisms,* as is the fear of insanity itself. But, mind you, the artificial world of phantasy that the psychotic sets up for himself appears decidedly real to him.

Depression.—There are those who take life more seriously than others, also those who get the blues readily when disappointed. Women are more disposed to depression than men and their physiological cycle may be responsible. Nor should it be forgotten that everyone is more or less subject to ups and downs and that this follows a fairly regular rhythmic curve and pattern.

Depression, however, is not *melancholia*. The latter, a psychosis, presents quite a different clinical picture; such patients worrying absurdly about some negligible transgression of the past, like stealing an apple, for which they are convinced they can never be forgiven. Depression, therefore, is normal. When despondency becomes psychotic it is extremely marked, of long duration, and shows delusions in addition.

Doubt.—This disturbance may become so marked as to lead to what the French call *folie de doute*, a sort of doubting mania. Here irresolution robs the individual of his will power and leaves him helpless. He is unable to make a decision and stick to it. Even after he does decide he begins to doubt whether or not he has done right and he may go so far as to try to undo what already has been done.

Especially in pronounced cases do people fear for the integrity of their minds. Doubt, however, is not a characteristic of the psychotic. The latter is really too sure of himself.

Anxiety or a *feeling of impending danger* does not lead to insanity. These are typical neurotic states and, of course, curable. Usually they are the outgrowth, in summary fashion, of a general, underlying neurosis that presents other symptoms as well.

Guilt and *inferiority* should be included as symptoms that often make people fear they are going insane. These have already been explained in a previous chapter. Although all neurotics are more or less suffering from guilt and inferiority, only when such feelings are pronounced do they become alarmed about becoming psychotic.

Various *errors* that we commit almost daily and definite *obsessions* and *compulsions* likewise scare people into the insanity bugaboo. Chapters VIII and IX, in detail, deal with these interesting mental factors.

There are various fears, besides that of insanity itself, that must needs be mentioned here.

To be sure, everybody is likely to become timid now and again. In fact, always to be fearless in every particular, even in the face of financial difficulties, critical illness or other impending disaster indicates lack of foresight and intelligence. It is also natural to be afraid to speculate in the stock market, to dive into shallow water, to run an automobile at breakneck speed and the like. Such fears are engendered by the instinct of self-preservation and are, as above stated, only natural.

Certain fears exist, however, which are decidedly neurotic. Fear of death may be placed in this category, likewise the fear of growing old, fear of the dark, the fear of poverty, fear of snakes, cats, worms and the like.

Then there is *claustrophobia.* It means fear of closed places. People who are harassed by this type of fear cannot feel at ease in a small or closed room, in a subway, elevator, and the like. They only feel safe when the place is large and the doors and windows are open.

An opposite, so to speak, to this fear also exists. It is known as *agoraphobia.* Literally agoraphobia means fear of open spaces. Such persons have a dread of crossing a street, a plaza or an open field; they also feel uncomfortable in large theaters or assembly halls.

There are also *aerophobia,* fear of high places; *misophobia,* fear of dirt; fear of a certain number and anything with which it may be associated; *anthropophobia,* fear of human society; *ailurophobia,* fear of cats; *hematophobia,* fear of the sight of blood, etc., etc. The list of possible phobias is a long one.

With regard to number fears persons exist who not only fear, say, 7, but all multiples of 7, such as 14, 28, 77, etc. There is a case on record where the patient became alarmed when the clock reached seven minutes before the hour and seven minutes after it. At these times he experienced a peculiar and indefinable sensation that something dreadful was going to happen to him, exactly what he did not know. Besides, whenever he ascended a flight of steps he would count them. When he reached the seventh step he would be in a panic. On the seventh of each month he stayed in bed all day because he was fearful of venturing out. Needless to say, the number 7 rendered this man's life a veritable misery.

Such manifestations are, however, neurotic in origin and, I repeat, they do not lead to insanity. They are merely symbols that represent something else; something the unconscious mind is trying to express. Psychoanalysis is the best method for all such cases.

In this connection it should be said that a psychosis is not scientifically considered a hereditary disease. It does not, for instance, follow the laws of inheritance set down by Gregor Mendel in 1865, and this is the ultimate test. Should you happen to find a case of psychosis somewhere in your family tree, whether near or remote, that fact in itself is nothing whatever to be alarmed about.

I stated in the beginning that if you fear you are losing your mind it proves that you are not in any such danger at all. To be afraid of anything really stands for a motivation to avoid it. If I fear becoming a dope fiend, whether justified or not, I avoid all medicines containing a narcotic.

Besides, in the last analysis, a fear (psychologically considered) embodies in a symbolic way an unfulfilled wish in the unconscious mind. That does not mean that a person who fears he will lose his mind actually wishes to be removed from reality and incarcerated in a mental hospital. Nevertheless, the unconscious mind plays with the possibility because, when insane, the individual is removed from his difficulties in the world of reality; he is excused; in short, he is allowed to escape without censure or blame. On the other hand, still more important reasons exist why, even unconsciously, he does not wish to be allowed to escape so successfully. A conflict between what insanity stands for (the wish to escape in a symbolic sense) and the wish to remain and fight it out resolves itself into fear. Through fear the conscious mind makes doubly sure that the wish for escape in the unconscious shall not be allowed to have its way. Therefore it may be said, in general terms, that when we are afraid a thing will happen we are doubly fortifying ourselves against its possible occurrence.

Although it is manifestly impossible to discuss, even briefly, every symptom that may drive certain persons into the conviction that they are losing their minds, it is to be hoped that, by consideration of the usual ones encountered, what I am pleased to call the factor of ignorance will be removed and consequently many people will be reassured. An old saying has it that what we worry over the most never happens. So be glad that you're not going insane and that your worst fears will not materialize.

Should this good news not make you glad after all, a final course still remains open. That is to consult a psychiatrist who knows his job; who, with specialized methods, sometimes with only a personal heart-to-heart talk, can chase your dread of losing your mind, as well as your other fears, helter-skelter. It is relatively an easy matter to assist you to live more contentedly with the world as well as with yourself.

Don't forget that every symptom, whatever its nature, has a meaning. It is a symbol that stands for something else—some repression, complex or conflict in the unconscious. The controlling mechanism of your entire organism, your mind, is sending out in its own way its S.O.S.

Your mind is trying, ever so hard, to make you better than you already are. It is endeavoring earnestly and persistently to adjust itself.

Chapter VIII

YOUR ERRORS HAVE A MEANING

DO YOU SOMETIMES FORGET FAMILIAR TELEphone numbers? Do you find it difficult or impossible to recall certain faces or incidents? Have you ever hesitated over the name of a friend or beloved one or called such a person by a different name? Do you overlook birthdays, wedding anniversaries and other important occasions? Are you in the habit of mislaying your hat, your keys or your glasses? Do you often oversleep? Do you make mistakes in writing, speaking or reading? Does your mind frequently go blank?

None of the faulty behavior I have listed may be true of you. Have not, however, similar errors annoyed or embarrassed you? Such reactions may appear trivial, even foolish; because of their repetitious character, however, they may become a downright nuisance, even give rise to grave concern.

Yet everything that occurs in the mind or that the mind causes us to do has a meaning and is purposeful. Especially is this true if it be repeated. No repeated error, whatever its nature, should be held to be insignificant. If you do no more than stub your toe as you enter a building, there may be a reason. Once a bride-to-be fell at the entrance to the church where she was to be married and sprained her ankle. She was rushed to a hospital and the ceremony postponed. The accident—if so it may be designated—was for her a blessing in disguise. She thought she wanted to marry but her unconscious mind not only reminded her that she did not, it actually prevented her from marrying.

No man, woman or child is wholly free from unintentional errors. We do and say many things that later seem strange and unexplainable. We forget what we should remember; we develop peculiar tastes, desires, impulses, likes and dislikes; we mislay or lose objects that are valuable; we suddenly divulge a secret we have protected for years. Then we ask ourselves: "Why did I do that?"

And well we may! *Every such error is a call for help* sent up by the unconscious mind. What you think with your conscious mind may be quite at variance with what you desire, feel and think within the *real you* which is your *unconscious* mind. The activity of the conscious is social, conventional, stereotyped in comparison with the unconscious, which is egotistic, primitive, instinctive and self-protective.

Discover the cause for your repeated errors and you rid yourself of such irritations, at the same time bringing to conscious recognition maladjustments in your inner emotional make-up, the removal of which should prove valuable in directing as well as smoothing the course of your life.

Should you *forget* a familiar telephone number at once ask yourself, Why? The reason undoubtedly is that deep down you do not want to make the call. I myself forgot the number of a hospital where I was to deliver a lecture when I was about to apologize for my delay. I had talked to that particular hospital perhaps a hundred times before. This was the first time, however, that I was consciously trying to do what unconsciously I did not want to do.

A colleague told me that when he decided to telephone his wife to say he could not be home for dinner he dialed three wrong numbers before he got his own. "It's because she always flares up when I'm detained at the office," he explained.

As regards one's *difficulty* or *inability* to *recall* certain faces or incidents, the unconscious mechanism is the same. The appearance of persons whom one dislikes or is jealous of, who have offended in some way or whom one fears, tend to be blotted from the mind. Incidents that by association carry a disagreeable emotional feeling-tone, such as an operation or a funeral, likewise fade from memory. Although the entire incident may not be forgotten, salient details are dropped out.

The more disagreeable an incident, the deeper is it finally repressed. A man may forget entirely that he once was jilted by a girl he deeply loved. The recollection of the pain attending childbearing never lingers long. Indeed, when we deliberately try to recall a harassing experience the mind may go quite blank. The unconscious mind always tries to protect the individual from again being emotionally upset.

Regarding *hesitation* over the name of someone we really know well, such an occurrence means that inwardly we bear that person an antagonism and that is why an attempt is being made to repress the name. A woman told me that when she is about to scold her daughter she invariably stammers. Another woman confided that, after a quarrel, she addressed her second husband as Vincent, which is the name of her first husband.

Be wary, therefore, of persons who continually forget your name, have difficulty in remembering it after being told, or address you with a name not your own. The same attitude should be taken if they should, but do not, remember having seen you before. There is likely to be some hostile feeling present. This may be of a personal nature or such a person may associate you with some disagreeable experience of his own not directly connected with you. To be sure, the real reasons for such social errors are seldom suspected.

For a husband to overlook his wife's birthday or wedding anniversary is proverbial. Here woman's intuition reveals her to be a good psychologist; she won't take "too busy" or any other excuse for an answer. She realizes that we never really forget what we want, with all our unconscious as well as conscious being, to remember.

A man who *mislays* his hat either dislikes it, wants a new one, experienced unpleasantness when last he wore it or he does not want to go out. And what you *lose* you may be sure you do not value, even if it be your wedding ring. Psychologists claim that we lose things because we want to be rid of them or the association they carry, but that we are unwilling to admit the fact to ourselves and actually throw the thing away.

An ardent admirer of the late President Roosevelt forgot the combination of the safe in which his Adjusted Service Certificate had safely been stowed away. He told me he had opened the safe only a week before Congress passed the soldier bonus over the President's veto, but that, try as he would, he could not recollect the combination since. After explaining the complex he had developed—that even if his conscious mind wanted to "cash in" his unconscious was still supporting the President—the combination of the safe came to him in a flash.

A certain man forgot to wind the alarm on several occasions, in consequence of which he was late for work. He also forgot his keys on two occasions and had to wake up his wife in the early hours of the morning. Twice he forgot to bank the furnace at night with the result that there was no heat the next day. In this case the unconscious was trying to tell him that he did not like living in the country although consciously he maintained that he did, for the good of the children.

A young man who was writing a Ph.D. thesis got into the habit of mislaying his glasses. Finally he lost them altogether. He admitted afterward that he "hated the job." A woman of my acquaintance always knows where she left her glasses when she wants to read a novel or newspaper but never when she wants to write a check. A widow who has been forced to sew for a living said: "I'm forever losing my thimble or needles or tucking away dress materials in out-of-the-way places."

Housewives may forget to season the soup after some difficulty with a member of the family. A psychiatrist told me that, after he had scolded his butler, he observed that the man forgot him when serving the dessert.

Oversleeping is, of course, an unconscious desire to avoid facing the problems of the day. It is a wish to blot out reality. One might call it an escape mechanism. Perhaps you have observed that you never oversleep when you have to catch a train or boat to go on vacation.

Mistakes in writing, speaking or reading are exceedingly common.

A doctor wrote to a former patient who asked for an appointment: "I hope you will not be able to come to the office at four o'clock Saturday." The explanation of this "slip" is understandable because the patient owed the physician a large amount for unpaid previous visits.

In my own case a patient once sent me a check for services rendered but failed to sign his name. The implication surely was no compliment.

A woman who wished to consult an attorney about a divorce wrote to him: "I have been married 22 years." But the second 2 had evidently been added afterward, indicating that probably she was embarrassed to admit not being able to make a go of it after living with the man so long.

In congratulating a successful political rival upon his election the defeated candidate mentioned his "ill-deserved victory." He meant to write "well-deserved." But apparently his unconscious disappointment could not be stilled despite the face he wished to put upon it.

Regarding errors in speaking numerous examples could be cited.

A social climber, in greeting a guest at one of her teas, said: "I'm so glad you came, Mrs. Vanderbilt." The guest's real name was Vanderburgh.

"Will you always bore me?" inquired a young lady of her lover. It is interesting to note that when the man showed he was hurt the girl insisted she had said "love," not "bore." And speaking of love, a schoolteacher revealed his secret to his pupils when on several occasions he called a child by the first name of the girl with whom he was infatuated.

In a crowded courtroom a witness let slip his opinion of the attorney for the opposite side by referring to him as a "liar" instead of "lawyer." So also a conceited astronomer gave himself away when talking to his class about relativity. He ended his talk with: "None of you can be expected to understand this subject." According to his notes he had intended to add: "unless you study hard." An expectant father revealed what was troubling him when, in commiserating with a man who had lost his home through foreclosure, he exclaimed: "What a great maternity!" instead of "calamity."

Mistakes in words often are the result of *condensation*, that is, two or more thoughts which the unconscious is trying to express separately, are rolled consciously into one, thereby producing odd combinations.

A woman who was talking to me about an intended trip to the lakes of northern Italy said: "I don't wish to visit Lavonia Bay." She, herself, was surprised, as no such place exists. Inasmuch as the trip was to be a honeymoon it was "love, honor and obey" that really was bothering her.

As regards reading, we often read what is not on the printed or written page and transpose, insert or omit words that reveal what unconsciously we are thinking.

For instance, a spinster confessed to me that, whenever she reads any word that is like "lady," "laddie," etc., she changes it to "baby." As an example of inserting a word not actually in the sentence a playwright, in reading the notice of a particularly sarcastic critic whom he feared, read: "Last night Mr. X's best play was produced," although the modifying adjective actually was missing in the review. During the First World War a mother skipped the name of her son which appeared in the list of casualties she was reading and would not believe that her eyes had played her false until later it was proved to her.

What might be termed *erroneously-carried-out actions* likewise are common.

In dressing for a formal dinner a man put on a bright red bow tie. His enthusiasm was self-evident. A physician who was supporting his sister in another city enclosed a statement "For Professional Services Rendered," intended for a patient, instead of the usual check, which he sent, instead, to the patient.

When, for instance, a usually efficient secretary makes errors in typing or shorthand, the excuse of fatigue or indisposition should be taken with a grain of salt. Resentment may have developed toward the employer or the work, or something may unconsciously be bothering her. Some years ago my own secretary often hit the *t* key by mistake. I discovered a young man by the name of Thomas was courting her.

In the case of the bride-to-be mentioned in the beginning the spraining of the ankle accomplished an unconscious purpose and was not serious. On the other hand, such purposeful accidents often *are* serious. I am familiar with a case where a man shot himself while cleaning his revolver and it is significant that this occurred after the market crash of 1929; furthermore, that he chose this particular time after neglecting the weapon for over a year. All sorts of self-inflicted injuries, especially when so apparently senseless, may represent unconscious motivations for escape or for self-punishment following guilt complexes. Nor can there be any question but that automobile accidents are often brought about by unconscious death wishes.

Psychologists speak of a *psychic censor,* that, like a policeman, is stationed between the conscious and the unconscious. It is this mechanism that is responsible for keeping repressed material repressed. In other words, what once disturbed or is disturbing consciousness is pushed away—"forgotten" the layman would say—into the limbo of the unconscious. However, if such repressions are vital to the individual they make the attempt to be recognized on the conscious level again and again. Since they were disturbing factors before, the censor tries to disguise them as much as possible. This explains why we commit errors and afterward wonder why we did.

It can frequently be noted that we *like* or *dislike* certain people for no apparently adequate reason. Here the explanation lies in our unconscious feelings; that is, some special characteristic, perhaps not at all well marked, connected with an unpleasant memory associated with another person. Despite what appears to be universal approval in others, a friend of mine disliked Fred Allen. He said that Fred's radio wit was crude, his puns corny, his style of comedy atrocious. And I know why. This man had a father who was cruel both to himself and to his mother. The father's voice had a sharp quality very reminiscent of Fred Allen's inimitable twang. I explained the unconscious reason to my friend about a year ago. Since then his antagonism to Fred Allen's program has entirely disappeared and now he is one of the comedian's most enthusiastic fans.

Note, too, your possible tendency to forget, misspell or change the names of your competitors, rivals or other members of your profession. Such persons you would, from the unconscious point of view, eliminate from the scene. Conscious training, however, interferes. The result is an error of some kind.

The unconscious even heeds the call of the physical. In other words, if an organ is affected a dislike may develop for tobacco, tea, coffee, alcohol and certain foods. Dr. Ernest Jones, of London, said that he usually placed his pipe in some corner where it did not belong and where he afterward could not find it whenever he began to feel the evil effects of having smoked more than he should.

Sometimes, too, you feel annoyed and you do not know why. Sit down quietly to think it out, however, and you will probably discover the reason. In *Caesar and Cleopatra* by George Bernard Shaw, the author pictures Caesar as upset, after leaving Egypt, by the thought that he had left something undone. Finally he remembered that he forgot to say good-by to Cleopatra.

Not only can you aid yourself by studying your own errors, you can likewise learn a great deal by observing the errors and attitudes of others.

If a person leaves an umbrella or any other article in your house, it is likely that he enjoyed his visit and would like to return. To neglect to write or telephone to someone, especially after promising to do so, probably denotes some measure of antagonism, although it may be mild. Forgetting to return a borrowed book may likewise suggest some form of hostility. Failure on the part of a husband to have noticed a new hat or gown is always a suspicious sign. To forget to greet another likewise warrants attention, as well as failure to mail a letter or carry out an errand for someone else. People who have difficulty pronouncing your name or are late for an appointment are trying, perhaps, to "high-hat" you. Those who don't look at you when they talk, refuse to accept favors, or fail to call you by your first name when you do them, likewise are not as genuinely friendly as they may seem to be.

It is by their errors that others reveal themselves to us and by our own that we reveal ourselves to ourselves.

Nor is it difficult to become proficient in this sort of mental detective work. Merely a little quiet introspection as well as honesty to face the truth are all that is required.

Errors such as I have been discussing cannot be classified as neurotic symptoms unless one stretches the elasticity of the term too far. My purpose in emphasizing them is to show how much, and in what manifold ways, the demands of the unconscious seek to make themselves known to all of us; how much they really have meaning.

Chapter IX

YOUR COMPULSIONS ARE CALLS FOR HELP

WE SHOULD, HOWEVER, CONSIDER ERRORS AS discussed in the previous chapter as mild types of *obsessions,* or perhaps better yet, *compulsions.* In other words, they obtrude themselves upon consciousness and force us into certain forms of behavior without our bidding, hence they are obsessive in character. Furthermore, we frequently must give way to them whether we will or no, even if we realize they are absurd, and these are the characteristics of compulsions.

All of a sudden, and for no apparent reason, you find yourself humming a tune, familiar or otherwise. After a while it begins to annoy you because it keeps repeating itself inside your mind without your humming it. In other words, a kind of mental humming occurs and it haunts you and you cannot get rid of it.

The cause of such a special brand of error again is to be found in the unconscious. Maybe it is the theme song of a musical show you attended, where you were accompanied by a person for whom you care a great deal. Perhaps the tune is of a lively character and the unconscious is trying to cheer you up. There are many possible reasons that, by association, may produce the obsession.

An illustration of an obsession more annoying because it seemed, from the conscious point of view of this particular man, to be more senseless, was the constantly recurring thought "mashed potatoes, boiled potatoes—mashed potatoes, boiled potatoes." It kept repeating itself for days until this call for help on the part of the unconscious was thoroughly understood.

Here the difficulty lay in the fact that the man had previously received a reprimand from his employer regarding his easygoing ways with the men who were under him in his department. "Don't be too soft!" the employer had shouted. "Be hard!" That very evening his wife served French fried potatoes that were burnt. "I should be hard with her, too," he mused. The next day the "mashed potatoes—boiled potatoes" obsession had been born. In other words, he could not make up his mind to be tough with his wife, after all, although his unconscious kept reminding him that he should.

A *compulsion* is really an obsession that carries an *impulse of action.* One feels impelled to do thus and so irrespective of how irrational it seems. One may or may not give way to one's compulsions. If one fights them down one usually experiences a sense of uneasiness.

Among the ordinary compulsions met with are the desire to go back to see whether the front door is locked, whether you have turned off the gas stove and whether you have put out your cigarette. Feeling impelled to touch gateposts or avoid cracks in the pavement, or to add up the numbers on the license plates of passing automobiles, are other examples. Then there are those who must look under the bed or open all closet doors before retiring. Indeed, a whole series of such acts may become obsessive and the individual in question may have no peace until he performs the entire ritual.

Making designs on paper while holding a telephone receiver or while in conversation may develop from an error into a compulsion, with the individual incapable of stopping himself from damaging his own and other people's desks, blotters, and tables. One such person would always roughly draw animals, such as pigs, chickens and cows. His deeply-rooted ambition was to own a farm. Another simply made up-and-down strokes with his pencil. These markings were symbols representing his lack of sexual gratification.

Compulsions may likewise be disturbing in character. There are those who feel impelled to smash electric light bulbs and shop windows. Even murderous ideas may be of a compulsive nature.

To be sure, obsessions and compulsions can be so severe, even torturing, that the individual himself cannot possibly work out their meaning. Such a person would then be said to be more than merely neurotic, that he was suffering from a genuine neurosis—a *compulsion neurosis,* if you will.

A patient was obsessed with the idea that whatever she touched somehow might poison, by the medium of contact, somebody else. Guilt feelings engendered by sex indiscretions of youth were the basic cause. She considered herself as one "poisoned." Therefore, although she knew it was impossible, she developed the idea that she could poison other people.

Another patient endured for years the compulsion of dressing and undressing three times before he felt comfortable in his clothes. Another had to walk around the block before he would enter his house. A third washed his hands with soap, afterward with alcohol, every time he touched a doorknob—a "dirt complex," so to speak.

Indeed, *thoughts* alone can become highly obsessive and undermining.

I knew a woman who kept thinking that an accident would happen to her children whenever they were out of her sight. The children were safeguarded well enough and this mother knew that the chances of harm befalling them were practically nil. Yet try as she would the compulsion persisted and caused her no end of heartache.

Young women frequently suffer from sex-thought obsessions. Of and by themselves these ideas about men are perfectly natural and normal. What makes them neurotic, however, is the fact that they keep crowding into the mind, forcing other ideas out. In some cases they actually prevent women from living a happy and efficient life.

Falling in love is a compulsion. To be unable to think of anything else but one's beloved can assume all the earmarks of a bona fide nervous disease.

Even conscience, as such, can become a compulsion. Always to have that intangible something obtrude itself into one's thinking and point the accusing finger of wrongdoing and guilt is a compulsion of the very first rank.

Conscience, to be sure, keeps us in line with moral standards and dictates what we shall or shall not do, what we dare or dare not do. For under the skin—and often not deeply at that—lies the untamed savage in each of us. We are afraid to let him out. We have been taught that he must remain buried and repressed.

When he does slip out now and again we naturally are tormented. We know we have done wrong and we accuse and revile ourselves. We may go so far as to consider ourselves outcasts, unfit to mingle with decent people and particularly with those we love. Such conscious mechanisms, you will agree, seem entirely exaggerated when held up to the cold light of reason and common sense.

Nevertheless compulsions are like that. Whether it be an ever-present and overdeveloped sense of conscience that keeps obtruding or whether it be the type of compulsion that forces a person to perform certain acts over and over again, the result is always the same, namely, mental distress.

And the cure always is the same, too—that is, the general method to be employed in each case is identical although the fundamental causes, even for the same compulsion in different persons, are different. For all obsessions and compulsions—whether of thought or deed, whether conscious and clearly defined or subtly disguised in symbolic forms—the cure always lies in digging up from the unconscious mind the complex or maladjustment that is responsible. Thus do you heed the mind's call for help.

A kleptomaniac, age seventeen, was brought to me when I was director of the Psychopathic Laboratory of the New York Police Department. This girl had a very comfortable home, was well educated, but was an incorrigible shoplifter. The articles she stole were of trifling value and her allowance was ample enough to have permitted the purchase of any or all of them.

A careful investigation showed that she stole only articles that had a point, like knives, scissors, needles, pins. She was caught taking an imitation diamond brooch, valued at $1.98, from a bargain-sale counter. Her room at home was searched and was found to be filled with innumerable trifles of similar kind.

The girl was Italian born. In Sicily she had always envied her brother's privilege of carrying a knife. Once her older brother stabbed a boy who had smacked her face. She was then ten years old. She admired her brother for this and wished to copy him but her parents taught her that girls must act subdued and refined. It was the special privilege of males alone to carry knives and stilettos and perhaps stab those who offended them. However, when she had a quarrel with anyone she would think: "If I were my brother, I could and would stab that person."

Later, when the family moved to America, she had quite forgotten the incidents and thoughts set forth above. The desire unlawfully to possess sharp instruments was still motivating her, however. Finally it transformed itself into shoplifting. She could easily have bought the articles, which were symbols of the knife or stiletto with which she could kill those who offended her, but the compulsion became master, so she took the unlawful way of obtaining these forbidden things.

Many compulsions and their analyses are less dramatic than this. Often, too, the explanation of the compulsion is not so involved and the unconscious complex, or cause for the compulsion, can be discovered rather easily.

Feelings of guilt and consequent self-punishment are often at the root of the whole matter, especially when the compulsions are torturing in nature. And in this connection I would like to stress the factor of compulsive sex ideas and acts in children.

It is fortunate that fathers and mothers are generally coming to recognize how important it is to try to explain sex matters to their children and, by so doing, to take the vulgar mystery out of it. It can be done so easily anyway. There are many books on the subject for children, and the approach to the realities of sex by means of examples taken from plants and the lower animals is admirable.

Every parent should try to win the confidence of his son and daughter to the extent that all sex questions, especially irregular sex practices, can be discussed frankly, freely and without embarrassment on either side. If the parents feel this is impossible then, at least, they should consult their physician or a competent psychiatrist who either will advise as to the best method of approach or will talk personally to the child himself. There are few children who do not worry about what is erroneously looked upon as "self-abuse" [1] at some period of their lives. When they give way to it without honest knowledge on the matter the seeds of self-accusation, convictions of guilt and inferiority are likely to be sown, and later in life unconsciously to torment the sufferer with some form of compulsion. This occurred in the following case.

Here was a man of thirty-eight, strong and healthy, well educated and capable, but holding an unimportant position in an advertising firm. His was a case where the conviction of being watched and the impulse to throw himself from a height were combined and marked. Wherever he went he would carefully observe people to see how he was reacting upon them. Especially was this true in social gatherings, where he would blush upon the slightest provocation. His place of business was on the fifteenth floor and he was afraid that he

[1] For amplification refer to Chap. V.

would jump out of the window. As if this were not enough, he suffered from insomnia, terrifying dreams and a terrific sense of loneliness.

The analysis revealed that this man's mother was unusually severe with him as a child. The father died when the boy was five. The mother became a dressmaker. Being of a nervous temperament, she punished the boy severely for the slightest naughtiness. It was not uncommon for her to lock him up in a dark closet and keep him there, despite his screams and entreaties, until he fell asleep. She also whipped him frequently with a leather belt belonging to the father. When she caught the boy practicing onanism not only did she beat him cruelly, she reviled him with unmentionable epithets.

Strange as it may seem, the boy grew to man's estate loving his mother and idealizing her more and more. She became kinder to him as the years went by. After a while he supported her and relieved her of financial burdens. The punishments and humiliations which he had suffered at her hands gradually were repressed into the unconscious and practically forgotten.

They were responsible, just the same—these repressions—for the symptoms I have listed, all really symbolic forms of self-inflicted guilt.

The blushing and compulsive feelings of being observed came from the childhood conviction that people notice it when a boy is addicted to sex habits; he was convinced, furthermore, that he deserved to be found out. He couldn't sleep after growing to man's estate because he continued to be tempted as when a boy. His dreams were frightening inasmuch as they indicated an upset, maladjusted state of the unconscious mind. Lastly, the impulse to jump from high places was an unconscious desire to do away with himself since he was so unworthy that he deserved self-destruction.

Compulsions are tricky things, and often most involved, beside being tormenting. The cause, however, can always be found and removed. The sufferer from compulsions can always be greatly helped if not completely cured.

The reason I speak guardedly about complete recovery here is because curing a full-fledged compulsion neurosis of long standing is one of the most difficult tasks to undertake in the whole realm of medical psychology. The difficulty lies, of course, in the fact that many persons with such deeply ingrained and habitual compulsions do not want to give the time necessary for a cure. For there are few indeed who cannot be improved, if not completely cured, provided they stick it out.

Tics and *habit spasms,* such as blinking the eyes, or mannerisms in walking, etc., may also be classified as compulsions. Even *stammering, stuttering, cluttering,* or *lisping,* that is not caused by structural defects, belong in the same category. Often the unconscious repression responsible is no more than a wish, for some specific reason, not to contact reality. In one man who was treated, months of "speech exercises" had done not the slightest good. In a few analyses it was discovered that he felt he did not want to live (contact reality) after his mother died, which was the time when his stammering started. After this unconscious repression had been made conscious, he quickly improved and finally was cured.

Probably no chapter on compulsions would be complete without a word on *superstitions.* These, to be sure, may become definitely upsetting no matter how much the individual in question recognizes their neurotic nature.

Although the psychology involved is not simple, we may say in summary that every superstitious belief carries with it an element of punishment which one is impelled to try to avoid. And why should one fear punishment? Because one feels guilty and deserving of punishment.

To put it another way, the source that is to inflict the punishment has, in your mind, become a rectifier of wrong, a symbol of some unknown power whose temper may not be trifled with. Such a power has decreed, for instance, that nobody shall become associated with the number 13 except upon pain of something dreadful happening. Since, unconsciously, you believe this power would punish you together with all sinners like yourself, if you disobey, you avoid 13 as much as possible. In other words, you subscribe to the ritual attending this superstition and you likewise find yourself superstitious in other ways.

It may be said, indeed, that the more superstitious you are, the more unconscious guilt you harbor and the more neurotic you are. Nor can you consider yourself a free soul in this respect if you say: "Of course, I'm not really superstitious, but why take a chance?"

In *Reader's Digest* for January, 1935, certain "pet economies" of well-known persons were listed that are amusing. These, too, are compulsions.

Bruce Barton hates "to see medicine wasted. Whenever half a bottle is left around the house by any member of the family, I always finish it," he says, "with thus far excellent results."

Kathleen Norris confesses to a "stinginess in the matter of

butter." Channing Pollock claims he could not make himself leave a hotel room with a single light burning. Ida Tarbell and Gelett Burgess won't throw away string, wrapping paper or glass bottles.

In conclusion may it be emphasized that the question is not: "Have you one or more obsessions and compulsions?" The question is how distressing is what you have?

If the compulsion does not especially annoy, simply leave it alone. Nothing of a serious nature will occur because of that fact. If it does annoy you can, if you wish, have it rooted out.

A great deal can be accomplished by oneself. For, after all, compulsions are habits of thought and action. To speak of them in a figurative but graphic way, one can think of these habits as water running along certain channels. Each time we give way to a habit the channel is worn deeper and wider. Each time, on the other hand, that we resist the habit we shunt the flow into other mind channels.

Although it may seem impossible to believe, even those with strongly vexatious obsessive ideas or with a definite compulsion neurosis were glad to be neurotic after their symptoms had been removed. In the analysis that was required to cure them they learned such tremendously valuable things about themselves they had never known before and, besides, so much about life in general. They now realize they could not have become so thoroughly aware of their assets as well as handicaps in any other way.

Chapter X

ARE YOU GETTING THE MOST OUT OF YOUR INSOMNIA AND DREAMS?

IN THE "JOURNAL OF KATHERINE MANSFIELD," the author says: "It often happens to me now that when I lie down to sleep at night, instead of growing drowsy, I feel more wakeful and, lying in bed, I begin to live over either scenes from real life or imaginary scenes. . . . They are marvelously vivid." She goes on to describe such an experience where she imagines herself on an ocean liner. It is night and growing late. Her father "puts his head in" and asks if "one of you would care for a walk before you turn in. It's glorious on deck."

If Katherine Mansfield could fashion such a beautiful mind picture, it is needless to say that she knew how to get the most out of her insomnia.

Yet insomnia can be an agonizing experience and develop fairly quickly into a habit that saps the vitality and makes the very thought of turning out the light a hideous prospect. It is a fact, too, that insomnia is a result rather than a cause, and that, as such, it can be overcome.

The person who habitually falls into the arms of Morpheus the minute he retires, and remains so the entire night, is a rarity indeed. As a rule, people are sleepless or restless sleepers now and again, some finding it difficult to fall asleep, others becoming fully awake after a few hours, then finding it impossible to sleep after that.

A change in weather conditions may be the cause, as well as increased humidity in the air. A strange bed may be to blame; too many covers or too few. Too little fresh circulating air may make a person toss about, or a rainstorm or a howling wind outside. An exciting day, book, movie, play or stimulating music may prevent one from sleeping. Overfatigue is a frequent cause, or working late when one is not used to it. There are also many physical factors [1] that may be to blame as well as a marked keyed-up state of the emotions.

Then there is the factor of irregularity of the hour of turning out the light. College students who for years have studied late often find it difficult in after years to fall asleep earlier. Of Jimmie Durante, the comedian, it is said that he never can sleep before two in the morning because he used to work in night clubs, and of the late Theodore Dreiser, a former newspaperman, that he frequently would awaken at three A.M. and remain fully awake until five.

The recipe for overcoming the physical and mental factors is, of course, to correct them. Regarding bad sleeping habits inherited from the past, keep trying until more beneficial habits are established. Regarding general rules that may be effective, a glass of warm milk, a few crackers, or a tepid bath; a cold shower followed by a brisk rubdown; deep breathing exercises before an open window; the reading of light or monotonous literature; listening to the radio; a glass of beer —any of the foregoing may work wonders with certain people.

[1] Consult Chap. XII.

Never, however, take to sedative drugs except upon the advice of a physician; nor should you ever become alarmed that your chronic insomnia will lead to insanity. Unconscious disturbances of neurotic nature may be the sole cause and those, to be sure, can be removed.

Let us, however, think of our "white nights"—particularly if they occur only occasionally—as having a meaning, as being still another way by which the unconscious tries to gain recognition.

What it frequently is attempting to say is that the sleeper's love life is not adequate. Such inadequate expression may pertain to whether the individual be married or single, whether he or she be of a philandering or promiscuous nature. Especially in reference to sex,[1] as such, may it be said here that sexual gratification is as much mental as physical.

When the individual tries to sleep and an attempt to blot out consciousness is made, then the repressions and conflicts that lie close to the surface, so to speak, have an opportunity to present themselves for consideration. That is why we phantasize so much when in bed and surrounded by darkness. The distractions of reality are reduced to a minimum. We think more honestly at such a time because we can introspect better. Many things become clear at night that were muddled during the day. That, however, is what prevents us from sleeping.

Despite the factor of losing sleeping time there is no gainsaying the fact that sleepless hours can be made valuable hours. That is why I ask whether you are getting the most out

[1] See Chap. XI, which discusses sex fully.

of your insomnia. Don't let it put you in a panic; don't roll from one side of the bed to the other; don't try to stop thinking.

Think until you find out what your *unconscious* wants you to think about. Settle that and you will automatically fall asleep. Then your mind will be glad and you will feel content. Suppose you do lose an hour or two? Even if you cannot make it up the next day, isn't it worth it if you have learned something about yourself that you never knew before, or if you have finally settled a problem that has been demanding solution for weeks?

Not that I am suggesting you carry your troubles to bed with you and make a habit of it. Occasionally, however, this is beneficial rather than harmful. The peace of the night allows you to think clearly.

And should you fall asleep and later awake, there is surely something important that is trying to escape from the unconscious. It may be that a dream is revealing an inner disturbance and that consciousness jumps into activity so as not to worry you. This self-protective mechanism concerning the relationship between insomnia and dreams will be understood more clearly after the discussion on dreams. Dreaming actually tends to prevent insomnia. It eases into the upper reaches of the mind repressions that must come out, without actually disturbing the dreamer to the extent of awakening him.

If insomnia has become a habit the chances are that a complete analysis of your unconscious mental and emotional processes is required. You have then reached a stage where it is impossible for you to get the most out of your insomnia by yourself, without outside scientific aid. Your repressions are probably deep-seated and of long standing. You cannot solve your problems by thinking in the dark, as previously suggested, in a conscious manner. Deeper probing of the unconscious is indicated.

Whether or not, however, you are of the type that cannot fall asleep, or the type that sleeps and then wakes up, you do sleep some of the night and undoubtedly you dream a great deal.

Try, therefore, to study your dreams. All have a meaning. Get the most out of them. They will shed a flood of light on your insomnia problem.

Dreams have always held a strange fascination. These weird mind pictures that visit us while we sleep seldom fail to captivate the dreamer's interest and, even centuries ago, they were believed to mean something. The Greeks and Romans accorded the dream great respect because they believed it originated from an outside divine power and had prophetic significance. But during the Middle Ages dream interpretation degenerated into the silliest kind of superstition. Only lately, one might say, has the dream come into its own, this being coincident with the advance made in psychology generally. For the past half century the mysteries of dream life have at last been solved and the dream itself put upon a scientific basis.

Nowadays it can be demonstrated that each and every one of your dreams, no matter how incoherent or sketchy it may be, is a definite attempt on the part of your unconscious mind to bring something to your conscious attention. In other words, understanding your dreams means knowing yourself as you never have before. What is more, via such enlightenment concerning your inner tendencies and capacities, you definitely can *make your dreams work for you!*

Indeed, the practical significance of the dream for the dreamer himself has always been stressed. For instance, when Alexander the Great was laying siege to Tyrus, the resistance of the enemy was so stubborn that Alexander was about to withdraw his army. But then he had a dream in which he beheld a satyr dancing as in triumph. The soothsayers declared that this meant the enemy soon would capitulate. Whereupon Alexander ordered a vigorous attack and conquered Tyrus. And then, of course, there are those two famous Biblical dreams that Pharaoh had concerning the kine and the corn, which Joseph interpreted as a prophecy, also in a practical way, that seven years of plenty would be followed by seven years of famine.

The "dream book" interpretations of our grandmothers' time—a remnant of the discredit into which dreams fell during the "Dark Ages"—were likewise intended to be more or less helpful to the dreamer. But reliance upon these unscientific interpretations has frequently proved disastrous. Only recently a business executive of my acquaintance dreamed that he was in a room where hundreds of birds were singing. "And what would you say that meant, my dear?" he inquired of his wife, with a twinkle in his eye. "That's easy," she replied, without consulting her pet volume. "Singing birds signify gain and success in a new undertaking." Whereupon this supposedly level-headed financier, acting upon what he must have considered a dependable guide, bought two hundred shares of stock because of an inside tip and promptly lost several thousand dollars.

When Aristotle in his treatise "On Dreams" (fourth century B.C.) stated that if, when dreaming, "one imagines one walks through fire and feels hot, it is because this or that part of the body has become slightly warmed," he really was breaking away from the then current notion that influences outside the individual himself were responsible for his dreams and, in effect, he was enunciating the first fundamental truth in dream psychology. That this view likewise embodies the personally helpful nature of dreams is nicely illustrated by the following dream of a friend of mine.

To use the dreamer's own words: "A devil with horns was sitting on the footboard of my bed and with long pincers he was placing hot coals all around me as though fearful he would not be able to keep the fire burning." The dreamer awoke, startled, and discovered he was suffering from a high fever. Whereupon a physician was called, the diagnosis of diphtheria made and lifesaving antitoxin promptly administered. Without this dream my friend would undoubtedly have had to endure a much more prolonged illness.

In fact, we often have dreams of this kind. I, myself, once dreamed that I was standing under Niagara Falls with my mouth wide open, and into it tons of water were tumbling without a drop being wasted. My body that night was calling for more fluid since I had eaten steak for dinner that had been oversalted.

Two thousand years had to pass before the moderns began to struggle seriously with the dream problem. Although such names as Schopenhauer, Strumpell, Hildebrandt, Maury, Kant and Havelock Ellis appear in the literature on the subject, they were more concerned with the purely theoretical aspects involved than with the practical significance the dream might possess. They quickly discredited the idea that dreams originate from sources outside the dreamer. What they finally proved was that the dream actually is connected somehow with waking life—usually with its disappointments—and that its real source may be organic, purely mental, or both, and that it always arises from within the dreamer's own mental processes.

A dream, to be sure, is nothing more than the continued activity of the brain while we sleep. During sleep, consciousness is blotted out but not the workings of the unconscious. The conscious mind, the waking mind, is merely an intermediary between the unconscious mind, which is our real memory, emotional and reasoning storehouse, and the world outside, frequently referred to as reality. The brain never stops functioning any more than do the heart, liver, kidneys, lungs or any other organ of the body. During waking hours the function of the brain comprises unconscious plus conscious activity. During sleep only unconscious activity is carried on. Some of this comes through in dreams. Some of it reveals itself in changed conscious ideas the following morning.

It has remained for Sigmund Freud actually to solve the mystery of dreams; that is, to unravel their causes and meanings. What's more, Freud's theories work; they are "pragmatic." By means of them not only is one able to understand oneself thoroughly, to discover unrealized tendencies, assets and handicaps—even to solve personal problems in the mental and imaginative spheres—but by means of them one can also find the causes for emotional, social, business and other maladjustments as well as the causes for neurotic disorders. Small wonder that nowadays psychiatrists the world over consider the Freudian approach to the dream the "royal road to the unconscious" and at the same time the most valuable single instrument they possess for the understanding, relief and cure of all kinds of mental upsets.

In summary, Freud contends that the dream always expresses an *unfulfilled wish*. That is, the wishes, the desires, the fulfillment of which is denied to us during waking life because of circumstances or moral, social or religious standards, are fulfilled for us, granted, during sleep. And, of course, we can see at a glance that the theory of Aristotle regarding physical stimuli deals, essentially, with body wishes.

If ever you have dreamed of a parent, child or beloved one dying, you may wonder how such a dream could be a wish fulfillment. A dream of this nature came to my notice recently and puzzled the dreamer no end. She dreamed she saw her mother lying in a casket; that was all. "Frankly, I do not think I could live without my mother," remarked the dreamer. "I am positive I do not want her to die."

Since the history of this person was known to me, the reason for the dream was clear. Briefly stated, this lady had never married because she had promised her father on his deathbed always to take care of her mother. The mother, however, consistently refused to live with a married daughter, hence three different proposals had been rejected by the dreamer. At the time of the dream, the dreamer was approaching forty. Soon it would be impossible for her to have a child, she thought. Yet, there was her promise and the impossibility of her marrying while mother lived. In short, one part of her make-up, the reproductive urge, managed to make its demands known in a dream despite the really sincere affection this woman bore her mother. Or to state it another way, a conflict of emotions existed in the unconscious mind which resolved itself in the dream.

The best way to test the validity of this modern wish-fulfillment theory is to study the dreams of children. In their dreams the wish denied in waking life is often clearly expressed and without disguise. For instance, a little girl of six asked her mother if she might lick the plates that had been used for the ice cream at her birthday party. Of course, the mother said no. That night the child dreamed she was a huge cat on the kitchen table lapping up plate after plate of her favorite dessert.

That the unconscious is always trying to help us, trying to heal itself, one might say, or better, perhaps, to adjust itself, the same as every other mechanism in the body, and that it can do so specifically, is evidenced by scientists, authors and creative artists generally who not infrequently find some knotty problem solved in one of their dreams.

A chemist friend of mine often dreams that he is working in his laboratory, puzzling over this or that, and—presto!—the solution he is after appears as if by magic. Indeed, he claims that even chemical formulas, actual equations, have thus been revealed to him. This man never fails to leave a pad and pencil on the night table when he retires. In the morning, he writes down everything he can remember that his unconscious mind was trying to express during the night, and should he awaken before morning the same procedure invariably is followed. He finds, as is true of dreams in general, that they tend to fade out quickly upon arising; so quickly, really, that one may not even remember that one has dreamed.

A dramatist I know also keeps track of the service his dreams may yield him. His imagination naturally is a productive one and he dreams, as he says, "the whole night long." No matter how fantastic his dream visions may be, they are studiously set down the next day and examined. "This helps one to get away from a too realistic plot construction," he remarked recently. "I see situations that are unusual. And not infrequently, when I'm stuck, I wait for a dream to show me the way out. Sometimes everything comes as clear as crystal; sometimes a plot is not so clear and I must perfect it consciously later on. My dreams, however, are more helpful than any collaborator or ghost writer possibly could be."

Some years ago an official in a department of police who was in charge of the detective division was psychoanalyzed. After the analysis he claimed that he, too, could make his dreams do his bidding in helping him to solve difficult cases. As proof of this he said he had looked in every conceivable place for a revolver that he needed to connect a suspect with a certain crime. "Then I dreamed that I had fallen down a sewer," he added. "In the morning I realized that an inspection of the street sewer outside the house where the crime was committed had been overlooked. I sent my men there and they found the gun."

It must be remembered, of course, that the unconscious mind is logical and directive as well as dynamic. Woman's intuition is proof of this, it being the result of unconscious thinking which she does not consciously realize. And the difference between a genius and an ordinary individual consists primarily in the fact that the former's unconscious mind serves him particularly well. A genius does not proceed in his thinking in a step-by-step and labored conscious manner. He gets results, arrives at startling conclusions and truths, by means he knows not how. But his mind only flashes and flares on the conscious level because of the preliminary, and often the entire, work which his mind on the unconscious level has done for him. It would be psychologically correct to say that such a person dreams continually while awake.

To be sure, we do not always dream as clearly as in the cases I have cited. Frequently the unfulfilled wish is disguised—that is, it is presented by means of *symbols*—and this is usually the case if the wish deals with repressions of which we are more or less ashamed, which are sexual or which are so strongly instinctive that they have had to be repressed again and again. The reason for such symbolization is that if the original wish thwarting—the repression or complex—were allowed to reappear in consciousness, the individual would be compelled to worry and struggle with it all over again. And that is why the solutions of scientific, play or other problems are not, as a rule, strongly symbolized; they have nothing to do with morals or other factors that may cause conscious embarrassment.

A dream I heard recently concerns thwarted sex strivings which happen to have been presented in an amusing way. Dreams seldom, however, are funny although, due to symbolization, they may be absurd, bizarre, illogical and improbable. Dreams are inherently serious because they stand for vital maladjustments within the mind proper, for repressions that the unconscious is trying hard to draw to the attention of the conscious so that they may be corrected.

In this particular instance a spinster dreamed that she was running about in the nude in an open space where there were numerous statues arranged along a path. People were approaching and she was trying to hide. Suddenly she spied a pedestal without a statue upon it and in a twinkling, jumping up, she took the pose of Venus de Milo, and remained undiscovered. The wish element here was a desire on the part of the unmarried woman to keep her primitive urges from being gossiped about. In fact, whenever her friends teased her she would stoutly insist that she was not in the slightest interested in men.

As an illustration of the repression of a similar type of instinctive urge that would not so readily be stilled consciously—the result, therefore, a more successfully disguised wish-fulfillment—a young married woman dreamed she was walking through a beautiful garden carrying a basket of fruit. Here the symbolism was plain, the basket standing for the womb, the fruit for the child. It happens that in this particular case husband and wife had decided that they couldn't afford a baby. The reproductive urge, nevertheless, was attempting to force its demands regardless of economic conditions.

Although most persons use the same type of symbols in their dreams it is hazardous to interpret a dream by symbols alone, without taking the personality make-up of the dreamer into account. It is possible, also, that the same dream symbol in two different persons may not stand for the same thing. For instance, wishes to escape some unpleasantness in reality usually present themselves in the symbol of taking a journey.

In analyzing dreams, however, I have frequently found that taking a journey meant quite the opposite as, for example, anticipated joy in taking a vacation or in meeting someone.

It is common knowledge that if you dream intensely you feel tired the next day. What has occurred is that the unconscious mind has been more active than usual and, instead of the nerve cells recuperating because of a regular lowering of functioning during the night, they have actually been working harder than during the day.

Particularly is this true of nightmares. Here the unconscious brain activity is exceptionally marked, with strong symbolization and heightened intensity, the reason for this being that the same repression—one highly emotionalized, like a definite fear or a marked disappointment in the love-life—simply will not remain repressed. Such nightmares call for a thoroughgoing review of the dreamer's life with special reference to his or her inability to express and adjust emotional urges. Often the individual, once realizing that the nightmare is such a call for help, can do this for himself since he now knows that his adjustments, such as they were, are not satisfactory to his deeper and fundamental strivings. Failing in this, as exemplified by a continuation of nightmares or frightening dreams in general, the services of a psychiatrist should be sought.

Incidentally, *somnambulism* is nothing but an intense dream, surcharged with so much energy that even motor as well as sensory nerves are activated. Incidentally, too, it is not dangerous—despite a popular conviction to the contrary—to awaken a sleepwalker while thus perambulating. Sudden, rude awakening, to be sure, may startle him. The fact that sleepwalkers seldom injure themselves is another proof of the self-preservation nature of dreams and of the unconscious mind in general.

Daydreams, so-called, involve the same mechanisms as night dreams. In these phantasies, when the conscious mind seems to break away from reality and ceases to be influenced by it, wishes are clearly set forth, without much, if any, symbolization. In fact, we speak of daydreams as a building of "air castles." In these instances, the unconscious desires break through before night comes and conscious repression is entirely eliminated.

I have frequently been asked, since sleep is a blotting out of consciousness together with its defensive and "on guard" qualities, and one learns so much about oneself by means of dreams, would it not be a good idea to anesthetize people? It is true, to be sure, that ether, chloroform, laughing gas and other drugs that anesthetize, even overdoses of alcohol, usually open up unconscious thinking, as it were; so much so that it fairly gushes out and creates the most fantastic mind pictures imaginable. The value of such productions, however, is negligible; first because the brain cells are not functioning normally since they are poisoned by the anesthetic, secondly because it is believed such drugs actually can and do, temporarily, break down the "myelin sheath" or protective covering of the nerve fibers, thus permitting nerve energy to jump across, in the manner of a short circuit, to the near-by nerves. The sum total effect, naturally, is an artificial mix-up of unconscious thinking, possessing no logic nor the possibility of being unraveled and understood.

The chemist and dramatist whom I mentioned previously are not altogether exceptional in being able to make their dreams work for them, either in whole or in part. In every case it is worth trying. To be sure, one's technique improves with practice. After a person has been psychoanalyzed and many of his dreams have been interpreted by a psychiatrist, it is always relatively easy for him to find the hidden meaning of his own dreams.

The way the analyst interprets a dream is to request the dreamer to let his thoughts drift aimlessly after thinking of each of the several important elements of a dream. The woman of the statue, for example, would have been asked to think of a statue, then what she thought of next, then next, etc. This is called *free association.* Sooner or later the dreamer's stream of thought becomes blocked, the mind goes blank. This usually means that a repression, a complex, has been reached. The thought at this point explains the symbol or part of it. Then the dreamer realizes what it is that he should not neglect, to which he should pay conscious and deliberate attention.

One time I, myself, dreamed of Santa Claus. That was all I could recall the next day. In following the free association method, I reclined in an easy chair, closed my eyes and thought of Santa Claus. First I could see him as the conventional figure children at Christmas adore; then my attention centered on his venerable white beard. After "white" my thoughts went to "snow," then Admiral Byrd's voyage to the Antarctic, then to "cold," then the cold of next winter. Then my mind went blank.

Persisting, however—in other words, trying to think hard and to push through this blocking—I came to the cause of my dream. My unconscious undoubtedly was reminding me to fill my cellar bins for next winter. When the dream occurred it was summer, when the price of coal is low. I had considered this before but had dismissed it from my mind because I was hoping the price might go lower still and because, frankly, I was resistive concerning the expense.

There are those who catch on to the free association method and can interpret their own dreams fairly accurately without even undertaking an orthodox psychoanalysis. Incidentally, it may be noted that dream analyses are being sought more and more each year by those who are not neurotic and who merely wish to learn more about the workings of their inner mental and emotional selves, to evaluate their mental assets as well as their liabilities. Indeed, dreams often bring hidden and unsuspected capacities to light. I recall vividly the case of a newspaper reporter who, in the course of professional dream analysis, learned that he had the makings of a novelist. Today he happens to be incapacitated by tuberculosis but earns a livelihood writing fiction.

It has often occurred, in the course of free association—used for the purpose of analyzing a dream—that the dreamer has at last remembered, consciously, something lost or forgotten. One person recalled by this method where she had hidden certain valuable papers; another remembered an important address; while to a third it was revealed why his girl friend was behaving coolly toward him. He had inadvertently failed to mention her birthday.

Dreams open up many possibilities, many points of view. New jobs may present themselves for consideration, business strategies may be devised, men and women may find out what they should do to gain or to hold the love of a member of the opposite sex.

"Never again will I poke fun at dreams," confided a man. "I needed money badly to meet a note due at my bank. I wondered and I worried and I got myself all wrought up. Finally, two nights before the dreaded date arrived, I dreamed of an old aunt of mine who is very fond of me. In the morning I paid her a visit and came away with the money." In this case the unconscious mind was more astute than the conscious.

If people by and large realized that every dream has a meaning and is more revealing than their own social conversation or facial expression, they would not be so eager to tell their dreams. Instead, they would take the time to think about their sleep thoughts and discover what their unconscious mind is trying to do for them. On the other hand, it is foolish to be disturbed over one's dreams, no matter how many wild animals may appear in them or how frightening they may be. Nor should one be upset if the mood a dream creates carries over into the waking state and is hard to dispel. Just remember that all dreams have a meaning and that this meaning is always a constructive one, aimed to assist you, to make you cognizant of the whole truth, without prejudice, concerning yourself.

You may be sure that in the not too distant future no person will be considered as educated, as prepared for life, or as capable of facing reality as he should be, if he has not mastered the technique of interpreting his own dreams.

In the past you may have considered your dreams nonsensical and your insomnia, whether occasional or habitual, a nuisance.

Are You Getting the Most Out of Your Insomnia?

From now on try another attitude. Get the most out of either or both. Nature did not create such reactions within yourself for nothing. Discover what nature is trying to do for you; assist it and make yourself glad.

As a neurotic you may not dream more than nonneurotics. Your dreams, however, hold precious nuggets of information that theirs do not. If you are not a strong wisher—and normals are not—you cannot have strong repressions and consequently rich dreams. And if anybody boasts that he falls dead asleep the second he hits the pillow advise him that this nonneurotic ability of his is not necessarily an asset.

Chapter XI

OF COURSE YOUR SEX LIFE IS FAR FROM SATISFACTORY

To find a person whose sex life is completely adjusted and gratified would be difficult indeed. Not that such individuals do not exist. They are, however, even among normals, exceedingly rare. In neurotics, on the other hand, maladjustments and dissatisfaction in the expression of the sex instinct are practically 100 per cent.

Nor is this to be wondered at. Remember that you, as a neurotic, possess urges of many kinds that are stronger than average. These would necessarily include the power behind the reproductive instinct; here, specifically, the sex impulse. Remember, too, that you never did fit in very well with any of the moral, religious and other concepts or customs that reality set as standards for you. And since reality itself is often contradictory, confusing and changeable, it follows that if there is one field of expression in which you are more likely to be upset than in any other it must be the sexual.

In a summary way reality, as interpreted by your parents and teachers, laid down these dicta: "As a child you will remain innocent of sex thoughts and practices. When puberty arrives and during your adolescence you will somehow learn all you need to know about the expression of your sex feelings. Again, somehow, the proverbial 'right man' or 'right woman' will step into your life and upon him or her you will project your sex desires by dreaming about and idealizing that person, by touching the lips, but no further. Then you will marry and your instinct will suddenly reveal to you what sex relationship amounts to, what it is supposed to signify, and how often it is to be indulged in. Likewise when you (a woman) become pregnant, instinct again will come to the rescue at the proper time to apprize you of all you need to know. In similar fashion will instinct be on hand to help you with the bringing up of your babies. Likewise when you (a man) find you are about to become a father, your idealized love will eliminate your sex appetite for about a year. And when both of you (man and woman) have been married for from five to ten years you will find that your sex impulses will gradually bother you less and less and, of course, the thing to do is to let them vanish."

Sounds perfectly idiotic, does it not? Yet I'll wager some of my readers have been brought up on ideas exactly like that, while others have had standards outlined for them that were more like these than they were different.

The modern child is not being brought up in so absurd a fashion. The nature and importance of sex is being taught even in the public schools. Parents are talking more freely about sex to their children. Books are to be had on the subject that deal with it in a scientific yet simple way and written for adults as well as children. Repression, sneakiness, guilt, shame and all the other evils that follow, when correct information on sex is withheld and when the individual is allowed to wonder and worry and castigate himself no end, may some day be a thing of the past.

But if you are a neurotic I'm afraid you did not have the

benefit of sex enlightenment bestowed upon you. Think back and you will recall how mixed up and troubled you were. Probably you are still mixed up and troubled right now.

It must be recognized that the sex life of the human species is not confined to a "rutting" season as in the lower forms, nor is it limited to the individual's need or desire to have an offspring. Few husbands and wives set out deliberately to have a child, while among the unmarried—whose sex lives are even more unsatisfactory than those of the married, so much so that the problem demands special consideration in all such persons—the possibility of being "caught" looms large both as cause for perverted sex ideas and practices and as a deterrent for complete sex gratification.

The facts are that the sex urge, being usually thwarted in its natural expression for some reason or reasons, becomes stronger and stronger. The facts also are that onanism, homosexuality, Lesbianism and perversions are indulged in much more than one might suppose. Nor need one be a psychiatrist to appreciate this. Statistics aplenty are available. But almost without exception those who are unable to marry and who carry on these abnormal methods of expression as some sort of outlet for pent-up emotion, or who marry and continue to practice them, do not realize that their make-up is intrinsically neurotic.

The same may be said of those who marry and find themselves philandering, or who are in some degree impotent or frigid; even of those whose sex interests wane quickly, or who never have been satisfied, or who suffer from the thousand and one possibilities that go by the name of "incompatibility" but that deep down are nothing more nor less than sex maladjustments.[1]

Nor is an unsatisfactory sex life, of and by itself, the whole story—that is, from the point of view of the pleasure or pain sustained by the individual mentally, emotionally or both. Repressed sex, irrespective of kind, may influence to a marked degree the individual's work, his efficiency, his happiness, his general social relationships, his glands and his health. So fundamental and primitive an urge as sex cannot be relegated out of existence, entirely or partially, without affecting the personality. So may it also be said, whether or not we believe the sex impulses to be the strongest that exist, that the man or woman who does lead a satisfying sex life possesses an asset that goes far in compensating for any nonsexual neurotic handicaps he may possess. A sexually adjusted person almost always is full of vigor, ambition and the joy of living.

Two general causes may be responsible for sex maladjustment. One is *conscious* inhibition, the individual deciding to refrain from responding to his instincts by an act of the will. The other cause is *unconscious;* in other words, the individual wants to respond but for reasons unknown to him it is impossible for him to do so. In all the conscious cases, however, an analysis of the psyche reveals that the individual, because of his childhood training, has been prepared for such conscious repressing. It always dates back, in the unconscious as well as the conscious cases, to guilt and shame feelings from which the individual usually does not fully realize he is suffering.

To state it another way, if you would only recognize that the sex instinct is not only a nagging urge but that it also is

[1] Consult Chap. XV.

not always "a pretty one" according to existing standards of civilization, you never would suffer from neurotic difficulties on this basis. Face the sex facts of your nature, whatever they may be, don't hide or repress them because nature is nature and there is nothing to be ashamed about, and at once your sex life becomes more satisfactory.

For instance, there are those who believe that masturbation has affected them mentally or physically for no other reason than that they *think* it does. There are those who feel disgraced because they experience for the same sex intense love that is sexual or borders upon it and they, too, lead a life of misery without ever committing an overt homosexual act. The same may be said of all other sex thoughts that deviate from the accepted normal.

Sex ability or inability lies primarily in the mind. Irrespective of unconscious influences, merely calling a spade a spade in regard to one's sex thoughts and feelings, and fearlessly, can wipe out many a neurotic tendency. Therefore, never feel guilty or ashamed about any sex ideas you may have, or had; never feel ashamed of what you may have done about it. The important thing is not what you have thought or done in the past but what you are going to do in the future. Somehow, all abnormal tendencies should be adjusted.

Here again, the factor of ignorance already referred to in this book, is pertinent. Few persons know what normal, average, sexual development implies. I have known men who believed since childhood that semen is "white blood," also that the penis is the prolongation of the spine and, through its canal, is directly connected with the brain. Many neurotic men feel completely exhausted after intercourse when, actually, the reverse should be the case. For the most part, men are woefully awkward as well as lacking in finesse and understanding as regards the sexual approaches they make. That a preliminary "preparatory stage" exists in which the woman is played upon, if you will, as on a musical instrument seems to be quite beyond their knowledge.

When we are born, Dame Nature must take care of the nutrition instinct first of all. She therefore establishes in the mouth area an *erogenous*, that is, a pleasure-giving, zone so that the infant will nurse as quickly as possible. If the child did not nourish itself it would die. At puberty, and for a like self-preservation reason, a second erogenous zone is established in the genital area. Nature, in all forms of life, goes to the greatest pains to foster procreation.

Now then, although every individual gradually develops away from his erogenous zones as other desires come into being, he never wholly divorces himself from them. When the erogenous zones are established it is understandable that the individual stimulate them; this being eating in the case of the mouth, onanism in the case of the genitals. That is why masturbation is, in a way, as natural as is eating and why it cannot be harmful unless excessive or unless the individual has been told that it is harmful.

It is also natural to overcome the habit of onanism. The goal of nature is not reached unless copulation be achieved.

The jump from autoerotic stimulation to heterosexual interest is not, however, a single one. There is always an intermediary step. In other words, after the boy or girl has been so wrapped up in himself he transfers first to a member of the same sex before he does to the opposite sex. He finds interest in bodies like his own (homosexual), before he finds interest in the bodies of the other sex (heterosexual). This interest may display itself in actual homosexual practices or it may be purely theoretical. This explains the "crushes" of adolescence and the interest in athletics where prowess of one body vies with that of another. It is only after this homosexual stage is passed that the sex urge finds stimulation and adequate gratification in association with the opposite sex.

Since the sexual impulse starts with masturbation, then becomes homosexual in character and only in the end is distinctly heterosexual, it follows that a person may not completely develop out of one stage into another. He may develop a *fixation* which holds him back from complete heterosexual expression. Such a person may continue to practice onanism or phantasize about homosexuality. But even if either or both practices be on a purely theoretical basis only, the individual merely wondering how "it might be," or being unconsciously so motivated without consciously realizing why, we find in such fixations one of the commonest causes for neurotic disorders.

Incidentally, it may be mentioned that definite arrests of development of this character, which usually are linked with glandular disturbances,[1] produce the actual homosexual and Lesbian, the male being vulgarly known as a "pansy" or "fairy." Such individuals are not neurotic, however, because they are quite satisfied to remain as they are. They do not suffer from repressions, guilt, shame or inferiority. They are not upset by sex conflicts because none exist. There is no urge present to be heterosexual.

[1] See Chap. XIV, in reference to the thymus gland.

To be sure, men and women differ as to the amount of male and female hormones each possesses. The average male has more female hormones than one might expect and still remains quite masculine in his behavior reactions. Many women have more than the average amount of male hormones characteristic of their sex. Each sex has at least some hormones of the other. Such differences from average, unless they be marked, do not appreciably alter the normal heterosexual urges.

It should not be thought, however, that I am advocating any form of sexual expression other than the heterosexual. This should invariably be the aim sought. If it is not possible so to adjust oneself, despite scientific knowledge—the truth—upon the subject, then a psychoanalysis is necessary.

Let it be pointed out also that a vast difference exists between *conscious control* and *repression.* Conscious control of sex thoughts and acts that do not harmonize with current standards may never result in neurotic symptoms if such control is not based on guilt or fear. In fact, some measure of such conscious control is *necessary* in order that the sex life be made as satisfactory as is possible for the individual who cannot control his environment as he would wish. But repression is another matter! Here one starts with the premise that one is wrong, that one must forget such wrongdoing as completely as possible. In such repression one finally succeeds in deluding oneself that the urge is not present, that the desire does not exist. But, as you already know, repressing an urge does not remove its influence. The repressed urge, when strong, may give rise to symptoms. In fact, the more you repress the more neurotic are you likely to become.

The *substitution* of strong sex urges is always possible, with results sometimes entirely satisfactory. This method is known as *sublimation.* It is a sort of idealizing of a basic, primitive desire. A spinster, for example, may have a strong sex and motherhood urge despite the fact that no man has asked her to marry. Sublimation here might be achieved through adopting a child, teaching school, having a few animal pets to love, doing social-service work and the like.

Lastly, it may be added that sex relationship, whether with or without marriage, never adjusted or cured a neurotic condition. The advice to marry is often given to unmarried girls who are neurotic. What always happens when such counsel is followed is that the already existing sex difficulties make two persons miserable instead of one. The problem of sex is not so simple as that.

But remember that you can neither neglect nor disregard your sex urges except at your peril. Whatever the trouble may be it exists primarily in your mind. Being neurotic you have undoubtedly harbored a wrong slant on the whole subject.

Chapter XII

TO BE SURE YOU'RE TIRED AND FULL OF ACHES AND PAINS

WHAT MAKES YOU TIRED? WHY MUST YOU endure nerve fag as well as physical fatigue? And if your body aches in addition and you suffer from malfunctioning of some particular organ even to the extent of pain, what is wrong? What is the reason and what can you do about it?

It goes without saying that here I am excluding actual physical disease such as organic heart trouble, tuberculosis, anemia, diabetes and other body disorders in which actual, structural changes have taken place in the tissues themselves.

Neurotic states, as such, no matter how mild or how severe, are nevertheless always *functional* and never organic. Your heart may palpitate, be irregular, "skip beats"; you may cough; you may suffer headaches, dizziness and nausea; there may be pain in the chest or throat; you may lose the power of your hand or leg; you may even go blind—yet, alarming though such manifestations be, they may be purely a state of neurosis. Such knowledge should make you glad.

If your aches and pains, your malfunctioning generally and irrespective of the organ to which it refers, are caused by neurosis alone they will promptly disappear when your neurosis is cured. On the other hand, if you do suffer from physical disease, your possible neurotic make-up should also be studied.[1]

Failure to appreciate fully the significance of the last two paragraphs accounts for so many people running from one doctor to another without being benefited. Sooner or later such persons are classified, sometimes even by physicians, as individuals who haven't anything really the matter with them, but who like to believe they are sick and be pampered because of it. They may even be called *hypochondriacs.*

Yet nobody wishes to suffer, and the neurotic with functional trouble referable to his physical make-up may experience actual pain which is not imaginary and which is as severe as if a cancer were gnawing at his vitals.

True hypochondriasis, to be sure, can likewise be cured, despite its existence for years. Hypochondriasis is a neurosis of the fear and anxiety variety. Such pronounced states [2] are merely obsessions, calls for help. It is a pity we can be so negligent concerning our fundamental needs as to allow the many physical upsets, found in a typical case of hypochondriasis, to develop.

If, however, you are suffering from excessive fatigue, fatigue without adequate or apparent cause, or you ache here or there and your physician says you are sound physically, don't for such reasons alone call yourself a hypochondriac. Your disabilities then are undoubtedly neurotic. But in true hypochondriasis it is characteristic that the patient jumps from complaint to complaint; first it is one part of the body, then another; he is in a constant state of alarm. He is depressed, sometimes

[1] For further clarification see Chap. XIII, "Don't Let Psychosomatic Medicine Alarm You."

[2] It might be well here to review Chap. IX.

morbidly so, about his own health; nor can he be made to feel reassured despite what a physician might say. The hypochondriac is, in effect, a case of severe neurosis, the removal of which demands specialized psychiatric procedures.

When physical symptoms exist in the average neurotic they are usually referable to one organ, possibly two, and the symptoms persist. The clinical picture is different from that of the hypochondriac. Besides, neurotics usually bear their symptoms well. The average neurotic, although he may complain a lot, stands a lot. Many are what nowadays would be called "bears for punishment."

I wish to point out, nevertheless, that you should never jump to the conclusion that your physical ailment is neurotic, or must be neurotic, because you know your mind is neurotic. You should first establish beyond possibility of doubt that your organic structure is absolutely sound.

Always select a competent physician, or physicians, who will give you a thorough physical examination, including laboratory tests, before you conclude that your physical disabilities arise from the mind.

I recall a case where a woman was referred to a psychiatrist for a psychoanalysis because the doctor claimed that the patient's pain in the upper right abdomen was not appendicitis but the "conversion symptom of a neurosis." Inasmuch as the surgeon who referred the woman was a capable man, the psychiatrist proceeded with his work. But the pain persisted; it grew worse. Then fever developed.

Although fever is not uncommon in neurotic conditions, this particular analyst, being himself an M.D., finally examined the patient physically. To his amazement he could feel the distinct enlargement of an abscessed appendix. The patient was promptly rushed to the hospital. An acute peritonitis was narrowly avoided.

Although I have stressed the necessity of ruling out all organic, structural causes for physical disabilities before the diagnosis "neurosis" is made, I do not wish to belittle the tremendous influence of the mind over the body. But to believe that every ailment you may suffer is purely mental is sheer nonsense. It is likewise unscientific to speak of the body and mind as though they were separate entities, each functioning in its own way and in entire disregard of the other. No, body and mind function as a unit, as one.[1] The physical affects the mental; the mental the physical.

That the minds of some persons have a greater controlling ability over their organs than the minds of others undoubtedly is true. Nor are all such individuals neurotic. Witness the power of mind over matter in the performances of Kuda Bux, the Hindu. Not only was he able, while blindfolded, with his eyes completely sealed with dough, to ride a bicycle without mishap through the traffic of London's streets, he was even able to walk barefoot over glowing hot coals without sustaining so much as a single blister!

Before we take up, however, the physical effects that can flow from the purely mental, let us consider briefly certain health rules which, if not adhered to, produce *fatigue.*[2]

Inadequate intestinal elimination is a prevalent cause for that "tired feeling" although individuals vary greatly in this

[1] This principle is emphasized in Chap. XIII.

[2] Gland factors that may be important in this connection are discussed in Chaps. XIV and XV.

respect. Most people eat more than they need for tissue repair and energy storage. Excessive drinking, smoking, dancing and night life likewise produce fatigue. Too little exercise, especially in the open air, is another cause. A rule frequently broken is not getting enough sleep, with the result that the tired one suffers from leftover fatigue from the day before. In this respect, too, individual differences exist, some requiring more than the average eight hours of sound sleep, some, especially the aged, less. Inability to relax or not taking the time to try to relax, especially for short intervals during the day when stress and strain are specially marked, or in the evening when the day's labor should be over, accounts for many cases of excessive and quick fatigue. Insufficient leisure, recreation or pleasure and lack of variety in mental and emotional expression are often causes for chronic fatigue or for its variant, a bored, disinterested attitude toward life. Lastly, the pernicious habit of carrying one's business and other worries home and into bed with one undermines the nerve and other cells of the body, prevents the recuperative forces from doing their work, allows chemical "fatigue substances" to accumulate and produces pronounced fatigue.

Since neurotics react in a faulty manner to reality in general it is logical that they should, as a class, neglect the essentials of right living as noted above. For such reasons alone, you may feel continually "washed out" and as weary on awakening as when you retired.

You, as a neurotic, use up more nerve energy than do other people. In fact, you consume your energy in unproductive and wasteful ways because you are continually thinking, thinking and thinking how you can straighten yourself out and be like the others whom you envy.

The neurotic, one might say, is forever stewing in his own juice. The problem from a physical point of view is really one of relaxation. He is unable to open up his nerve junctions (synapses) so as to give his nerve cells a chance to rehabilitate themselves. He is constantly in a state either of fight or flight, usually the latter, in a figurative way of speaking. After a while his glandular system [1] likewise is affected, especially his adrenals. Then he designates himself correctly when he says he is "all in."

Let us now consider, from the structural side, how complicated the brain is.

Dr. C. Judson Herrick, in a paper read before the American Association for the Advancement of Science, stated that he estimated, after extensive research, that the nerve cells in the brain number from ten to fourteen billion, and that their fibers which connect with other cells run to a stupendous number—something like fifteen million ciphers placed after the figure one.

What is more, it has definitely been proved that nerve energy is electricity. Such mind currents have been drawn from the brain and recorded. The greater the amount of thinking there is, the greater the degree of emotion, the greater also is the amount of electricity used. What actually makes thought or emotion, what the exact nature of the electrochemical processes involved is, still remains a mystery.

In addition to the enormous amount of brain cells it must

[1] Consult Chap. XIV.

be remembered that the brain has another essential function besides that of giving rise to thinking and feeling. Every tiniest piece of tissue situated anywhere in the body is connected, via special nerves, or in an indirect manner, with the brain proper. The brain, therefore, is the coordinating organ of the entire system. It is like a highly-sensitized, automatic, electric switchboard.

It is not to be wondered at, therefore, that the mind, as such, can and does influence the body in so commanding a manner. To state it differently, the needs and demands of the mind can, and frequently do, manifest themselves in physical disturbances.

Unless one is used to seeing cases where aches, pains and almost any variety of physical disorder are nothing more than different forms of calls for help—as obsessions are—on the part of the mind, it is perhaps difficult to believe that such strange manifestations can occur. Yet there are rather few neurotics, comparatively speaking, who are not troubled by some physical upset that may be serious or merely irritating. That is why the title of this chapter is "To Be Sure You're Tired and Full of Aches and Pains."

Nausea and vomiting, for example, are frequently encountered. They may be nothing more than symbolic expressions—in the physical sphere but produced in the unconscious mind—of a desire to rid the individual of complexes that are getting out of hand and are becoming too annoying; or the nausea and vomiting may represent a repression or repressions linked with shame and disgust.

Here, as in most symptoms that are converted complexes, it is as if the unconscious said: "If I can't get recognition in the conscious mind so as to have this troublesome thought removed, then I will get conscious recognition by means of a roundabout route, namely, a physical sickness."

In a similar way a choking sensation in the throat may represent, symbolically, self-punishment; headache may be produced by conflicts between opposing instincts or wishes; dizziness may stand for escape from reality; heart trouble for fear of the future; self-pity may represent an urge to self-destruction or a symbol of thwarted love, etc. The familiar functional paralysis of writer's cramp often is nothing more nor less than a sign that, although the conscious mind wants to write, perhaps in order to make a living, the unconscious is saying "no" for even better reasons.

A case that neatly illustrates to what extent the unconscious will go to make its needs known, concerns a navy man who, during the war, suddenly went stone blind. He was on a submarine chaser at the time; he could not account for his disability; nor, after he had been brought ashore to a hospital, could eye specialists find a single bit of pathology referable to his eyes. In other words, the lenses, the optic nerves, the muscles—the entire eyeballs—were anatomically normal. Yet the man could not see; could not even distinguish light from dark!

An analysis of his mental process, however, revealed the cause for this devastating physical calamity. In fact, the trouble when found was simple. Here was a man who had voluntarily enlisted in the Navy before he was drafted in the Army. "I wanted to do my bit without being forced," he explained. Nevertheless, despite his ego strivings (his ego instinct), the self-preservation urge, which he had repressed, tried to stop him from risking his life. It failed, to be sure, because the man found himself on a submarine chaser, assigned to dangerous duty.

How then could the self-preservation urge, now in conflict with the ego urge, assert itself? One way at least was to render the man sightless. Then he would be taken off duty and his life safeguarded. Nor could anybody, nor he himself, then point the accusing finger and cry "Coward!"

To complete this history, it may be said that when the psychiatrist was able to piece together all the data gathered in the analysis, when he was able to explain to the patient that his warring ego and self-preservation instincts had, so to speak, agreed to compromise their differences by causing his blindness, thus preventing him from endangering his life, a ray of hope lighted his face that was marvelous to behold.

"Then I ought to be able to see?" he cried.

"Certainly. Take off those bandages and prove it to yourself."

You may finish this story any way you like. Needless to add, *that* sailor man, although he had suffered one of the most severe of neuroses, was the happiest man in the world.

Chapter XIII

DON'T LET PSYCHOSOMATIC MEDICINE ALARM YOU

IN DISCUSSING YOUR ACHES AND PAINS AND THE neurotic fear that you may be suffering from an actual organic disease, I emphasized that in such cases the organs are physically sound. I stated, also, that organic disease, of and by itself, may produce nervous manifestations, so much so that whatever the laboratory tests, X rays or other diagnostic procedures reveal, the patient complains of more symptoms than these justify.

Your neurotic make-up—specifically your *emotions*—can, however, be responsible to an appreciable degree for actual changes in organic structure. In an indirect way the emotions interfere with the proper functioning of certain organs and trouble results.

Nowadays, therefore, the thorough surgeon and internist is not satisfied when he discovers the existence of pathology (physical diseases); he no longer thinks his work is done in arriving at a diagnosis when he has employed all necessary or available laboratory aids. Such a doctor, in addition, inquires into the emotional life of his patient. He wants to find out if factors exist that somehow contributed to the physical abnormality discovered or that may retard the progress of the patient or his cure. If his patient is organically ill, the doctor wants to know how much the feeling reactions and general outlook of the man's case tie up with his physical condition. In other words, to what extent do his emotions make the man sick?

That is what is meant by *psychosomatic medicine.* It is a ponderous name but it stresses simply the fact that the mind ("psyche") and the body ("soma") constitute a single unit, neither one being independent of the other. The coining of the word psychosomatic is really a belated acknowledgment on the part of the medical profession at large—accustomed too long to evaluate all diseases in terms of the organic alone—that the mind, after all, is a powerful factor in physical and physiological, as well as mental, well-being.

The Medical School of Columbia University is now conducting the first Psychoanalytic and Psychosomatic Clinic in the country. At the Neuropsychiatric Center in Boston a so-called Thought Clinic devotes itself to adjusting patients to their social and emotional difficulties. This is only the beginning.

When we are talking about psychosomatic medicine, remember that we are considering actual organic disorders that may not seem to be associated with any emotional factors at all but which, nevertheless, are. The emotional centers affect the functioning of the organs, and these, in turn, may produce changes in structure. More than half of all the cases seen by the general practitioner present emotional problems of one kind or another that should not be overlooked. Unless these are corrected the doctor cannot hope adequately to cope with the physical disabilities found.

To the gastrointestinal specialists come scores of men and

women with stomach or intestinal upsets, including ulcers and colitis. The acidity of the stomach is appraised as well as its motility and emptying ability, test meals are given, the fluoroscope and X rays are brought into use, the patient is put on a diet and medicated. As a parting blessing the doctor pats his patient on the back and says, "Take it easy now and don't worry."

But the trouble is that the patient is unable to take it easy and he continues to worry. Maybe he is working too hard because he fears competition and the loss of his job. Maybe he's got a nagging wife. It could be that he's got another woman on his mind, or that he thinks his wife is unfaithful or, at least, has lost her love for him. Maybe he is worrying over the welfare of his children.

Well, such a man never can be cured of his ulcer or whatever it may be until his emotional conflicts are brought to the surface, talked out and adjusted. Even if he gets over one ulcer he is almost certain to develop another if his basic neurotic disposition is not changed.

The same may be said of "heart trouble," a term that covers such a multitude of sins. Here is an organ that the patient actually hears functioning. Merely centering his attention on its beat, or taking his pulse, increases it.

The heart specialist makes an electrocardiogram besides examining the offending organ in the usual way, and either tells the patient that his heart is sound or that there is something organically wrong. How often, however, does he inquire into the patient's emotional make-up and what makes him emotional? Whether the heart disorder is organic or functional, improvement or cure cannot be hoped for unless disturbing emotional factors are removed. These concern the way the mind works, the way the patient thinks, feels and behaves.

Many abdominal and other operations are performed, and of necessity, where the patient in the end seems no better off than before. Even in organic heart disease the final collapse of the organ may be postponed and the patient complete his normal life span provided that devitalizing mental stress and strain are removed.

A woman was "opened up," as she phrased it, three times because of intestinal obstruction. Had the aid of a psychiatrist been enlisted, once would have been enough. The "chronic appendix" diagnosis is a case in point. Perhaps the patient is just as well off to have it out, but why should his complaints persist afterwards? Indeed, there are cases that may be classified as "postoperative neurosis," and with propriety. The surgeon finishes his job and does it well, but he does not usually realize the psychic effect his assault on the body of the patient may produce. People become alarmed over high blood pressure and are treated medically for years when all that is necessary, perhaps, is the change of a job or a way found to pay the mortgage on a home.

Asthma, hay fever, migraine, skin rashes and allergies of various kinds, eczema, nervous indigestion, diabetes, ovarian and menstrual dysfunctioning, frigidity and impotence, tuberculosis, infectious diseases and the common cold, unexplained fever, backaches, headaches, dizziness, weakness, fatigue, as well as many other organic disorders—each may have a psychosomatic story all its own. Exactly how and why certain types of emotional shocks and conflicts affect certain parts of the body and not others is still a matter for further research. Generally speaking, however, hostility toward parents, deep resentments, feelings of insecurity, convictions of being "unwanted" or of "not belonging," conflicts regarding love, reluctance to reveal emotion to others and an attitude of not being willing to face and cope with reality—although possibly unable to because of repressions dating from childhood—are the chief causes.

If your doctor examines you and says, "I can't find anything organically wrong with you," raise the question whether your emotions may not have something to do with your condition—if you are not neurotic. Should he say you are suffering from an organic ailment, inquire what steps you should take to regulate your life in order to speed your recovery. Ask specifically whether the latter is not actually the crux of the entire problem.

Although psychoanalysis is undoubtedly the most thorough way of reaching the inner emotional self, thereby straightening out the psyche which, in turn, affects the physical organs favorably, treatment of such a kind need not consume months. All that may be required are a few searching talks at the hands of a man who has studied the mind and its influences, who is understanding, who does not sit in judgment on your case and who does not scold. With him you must be frank, feel confident and unafraid.

Do not think, of course, that every emotional maladjustment, even if severe, will lead to organic change, if only to a minor degree. Usually it does not. Merely be on the alert to see if it does; best of all, remove your neurotic tendencies and take no chances.

At any rate, psychosomatic medicine should not be terrifying. Its advent is merely another step in the forward march of science to help you.

Chapter XIV

ARE YOUR GLANDS ON FRIENDLY TERMS?

WHAT MAKES US THINK THE WAY WE DO? Why is it one person acts so differently from another? How can we explain the striking differences in individual feeling reactions?

A crowd is waiting at the intersection of a busy street. There may be fifty people expectantly watching for the red signal to turn to green. Three of them become impatient; they think they see an opportunity to cross; they run. A car suddenly bears down upon them. The driver jams his brakes.

A dodges, keeps his head, quick-wittedly avoids another car, gains the sidewalk in safety. *B* stands stock-still, apparently expecting to be struck, accepting the situation with calm and resignation. *C* hesitates, wavers, jumps forward and backward, then runs head-on right into the car. The impact knocks him unconscious. The driver hastens to his assistance and *C* finally revives. Recognizing the driver, he flies into a rage, uses the vilest language and plants his fist on the surprised driver's jaw.

Temperament, habit, environment, heredity, training, personality—which? The McDougallians cry "*Instinct!*" "No," retort the Freudians, "*complexes!*" "Wrong again," shout the behaviorists, "can't you see it all depends upon the *conditioned reflex?*"

Haven't we got the explanation yet why some of us, like A,

are keen, intelligent, quick on the trigger, rational, common sense? Don't we know why, like *B*, we may be slow, stolid, reserved, fatalistic? Is there no unanimity of opinion about people who, like *C*, are unstable, fiery, vituperative and maniacal?

And then, regarding other attributes. How does it happen that one person succeeds and another fails when it is obvious the reverse should be the case? What makes for contentment and discontent? Wherein lies the basic cause for achievement? What's wrong when our love lives remain bottled up and longing? Why do we lie, deceive, become unfaithful, steal, murder, sometimes despite the fact that we fight against such impulses with every available grain of energy?

Is there neither rhyme nor reason about this sphinxlike riddle of human behavior? Cannot modern science find an Oedipus to solve it? Just where, and in what, are we to seek for the why and the how and the wherefore?

One must admit that the Freudians have had the best of it thus far. At least they have received the most publicity. That psychoanalytic probe of theirs has penetrated deeply. Apparently it has reached hitherto inaccessible places. It has explored the disguised and mysterious reaches, even the darkest and most offensive wellsprings of human conduct. Relentlessly that probe has pierced pride, sham, pretense, bluff, culture, refinement, and exploded them like so many toy balloons.

The psychoanalytic theories based upon the primitive, unconscious self in conflict with the socialized and standardized world of reality, the repressions caused thereby, the complexes built up as a result, the handicaps thus established—these interpretations of individual differences have gone a long, long way in explaining what hitherto appeared hopelessly inexplicable. And the explanations have worked! That's the best of it. People have been changed and helped. Not always, of course. On the whole, however, psychoanalytic theories have proved pragmatic, which is more than can be said of the others.

To be sure, it has not been a flattering investigation. The psychoanalytic probe has hurt. It has shown us up as a pretty shoddy lot. Sex? Sex aplenty! Yes, often skulking, sordid, perverted sex and from places surprisingly unexpected. But at least, and at last, sex has fearlessly been roped and thrown; it has been dragged up out of its hidden lair in the unconscious and into the light of day. That's something. We are not so afraid of sex as before. Generally speaking, frankness has had a cleansing effect. We have been revealed for what we really are, all of us, without favor or exception. That is what the psychoanalysts claim. They say our very soul has been dissected and laid bare.

Whether right or wrong, pretty thorough stuff at any rate, don't you think? Can anything more be said when these researchers of the psychic insist that as adults we are motivated by stimuli impinging themselves upon the mind while we are waiting to escape from the mother's womb? Certainly it is not possible to go back further than that!

But we haven't got the whole story after all. Not yet! Our individual differences in thinking, feeling and action seem to be explained, but the truth is not always what it seems. When all is said and done the various schools of psychology have been talking psychology. It's the *mind* that has captivated and fascinated them.

What about the *body?* Has sight of that been lost in the scuffle? We must not forget that the ancients did not believe the soul was lodged in the mind. No fools were they, either. They located the soul in the pit of the stomach.

Anyway, here enter the physiologists!

And with the physiologists enter the *thyroid,* the *adrenals,* the *pituitary,* the *pineal,* the *thymus* and the *sex glands!* These are the famous endocrine glands, also known as the "ductless glands" and the "glands of internal secretion."

Here, indeed, is a troop to conjure with; an all-star cast if ever there was one. Each a principal, each a leading player, each an absolutely indispensable factor in motivating, shaping and determining the drama of human destiny.

Laying bare the secrets of the soul—eh? Yes, that's a pretty good job. Let us give the devil his due and include the psychoanalysts. But these physiologists and their endocrine glands! These Stanislavskys and their Moscow Art Theater players! There is no use trying to force the metaphor. The physiologists have undoubtedly gone the psychologists a step further. That's the marvel to emphasize. They have taken the step which some day may explain of what stuff the soul actually is made!

Inorganic chemistry enacted a compelling role in bringing industry where it is today; organic chemistry revolutionized agriculture; now physiological chemistry is throwing the spotlight upon human conduct.

Remember what A did when suddenly confronted with the automobile? He made the proper dodges and won. Each school of psychology would have given him 100 per cent plus on this particular reaction. I can hear Freud himself declaring that *A*'s analysis would scarcely be worth doing. So average a reaction could only come from a most prosaic and commonplace person. And an automobile bearing down upon you may be a sex symbol at that, you know, especially if you dream it. But A did not dream it. It was an actual fact of reality for him. Certainly it was a perfectly normal act to escape so adroitly at the moment, sex or no sex.

And the physiologists? What of them? "All glands in balance," would be their verdict on A. And, of course, quite uninteresting.

Let us examine *B*. He it was who stood still, docile and inactive, ready and waiting to be hit. "Introverted, shut in, repressed, day-dreaming," the psychoanalysts would declare. "Suffering from a marked inferiority complex with shame and guilt accompanying. Self-accusatory and self-depreciative because of infantile sex transgressions. So unworthy he felt he ought to be killed."

The physiologists? "Deficient thyroid. In other words, a hypothyroid state. Didn't you notice how short, fat and pudgy he was in addition to that marked mental and motor sluggishness? A few tablets made from sheep, hog or goat would have brought his gland system back into balance. Let us hope he takes them before he attempts to negotiate the traffic again."

Now C. He got entirely rattled, knocked himself down and out, later flew into a rage and attacked the chauffeur. "Sex hunger," the Freudians would declare. "Always keyed up and irritable because of it. Undoubtedly suffers from insomnia and when he does sleep his dream life must be productive, distorted and possibly frightening. Automobile unquestionably has sex significance for him. The mechanical principle involved is that of the piston in the cylinder; besides, an automobile is a self-propelling machine and suggests onanism. At any rate, to C the car is both enticing and menacing at one and the same time. His feeling toward it is 'ambivalent.' His falling unconscious was a symbolic escape. Attacking the driver suggests a homosexual defense, but of that one cannot be absolutely certain. A thorough analysis is indicated to clear up this point. It might take months. But then, the man needs an analysis as much as food. He is heading for a complete nervous collapse."

And again the physiologists? "As obvious a case of deficient (hypo-) adrenal functioning as one could wish to see. The adrenal glands have to do with maintaining the tone of the muscles and nerves in emergencies. C used up his adrenal reserve in attempting to run across the street and in trying to make up his mind what to do when he found himself trapped. That's why he fell unconscious. During that brief interval his adrenals worked overtime and another reserve supply was furnished. The quick temper and the pugnacity is typically an adrenal reaction. This man also needs glands and it might be better to administer them by 'hypo' and put him to bed."

Does this account amuse you? Do the views of the leading psychological school as compared with that of the physiologists seem far-fetched and possibly even contradictory?

As a matter of fact, they are neither one nor the other. Each has reasoned the particular behavior under consideration quite logically and according to Hoyle. One uses the method of mind approach; the other takes the physical route. *Both* are valid. Both can be turned to the benefit of *B* and C.

Regarding the adherents of the McDougall school and those that follow in Dr. Watson's footsteps, well, I'm afraid we shall have to drop them here. Instincts and conditioned reflexes would not do *B* and *C* much good.

But let us not permit diverse opinions upon an identical problem to upset us. Nowadays we must constantly expect to have our pet theories knocked into a cocked hat. We think we know something today; tomorrow we find that that much ignorance won't get us by a Binet test or one of Edison's former questionnaires.

In this instance, though, we are lucky. We are not compelled to snub any of our old relations in order to embrace these new members of our mental family. Your mother and father fixations and your inferiority complexes can still remain friendly with your endocrine glands. In fact, you will find that intimate acquaintance with all of them can only redound to your own personal advantage.

Glands are not new, of course. When I tell you that one of them, the *pituitary*, situated at the base of the brain, is supposed to be the remnant of a third eye which prehistoric lobsters boasted of, you will obtain some idea of the number of years those glands of ours have been in existence.

The Chinese employed glands for physical ailments hundreds of years ago. They dried frogs and newts, powdered them and tried them for epilepsy and heart disease. They also employed canine orchitic extracts for the treatment of obesity. Decoctions of lizards, toads and spiders had been used blindly, but with salutary effect, for goodness knows how long. Recently, scientific investigations revealed that the skins of these beasties harbor tiny adrenal glands which manufacture an appreciable amount of adrenalin.

The really new thing about glands is a recognition of the way they affect human nature, especially our intellectual and emotional lives. It is no exaggeration to say that we think, act and feel, not only with our *brain,* but also with our *glands!* The way these glands interlock and cooperate with thc brain pan is a piece of physiological-psychological machinery than which nothing could be more marvelous.

Suppose we examine more closely into the hidden mechanisms that made C behave the way he did. I am sure you consider him the most interesting fellow of the three. And I feel certain you will agree further that a dovetailing of his psychoanalytic explanation with that of his gland interpretation is interesting.

When C found himself confronted by the automobile he realized what was happening through his sense organs, especially those of sight and hearing. With a travel speed greater than that of light the message of danger was at once flashed along nerve paths to the spinal cord and from the spinal nerves to the autonomic nervous system in front of the cord. Again with kaleidoscopic speed the message was shunted over to the adrenal glands, to each of them, since there is one seated on top of each kidney. Immediately the adrenals let go their reserve supply of adrenalin which, circulating in the blood, activated the liver. The liver responded by pouring into the blood its stored-up sugar, otherwise known as glycogen. This glycogen stimulated all the muscles and got C ready for *flight or fight.* There you have it in a nutshell.

This is what occurs between the brain and the glands and

the organs of the body in every emergency. If you suddenly came upon a tiger running loose in a park, that is what would take place. If you have a heated quarrel with your husband or wife or sweetheart, it's the same thing. Always the brain prepares the adrenals, which prepare the muscles, for flight or fight.

And which you do depends upon your adrenal reserve and your unconscious complexes!

If the automobile had not been a sex symbol for *C* he might have used his slight adrenal reserve in propelling his legs faster. In consequence he probably would have succeeded in escaping the danger as well as *A* did. But automobile was his complex. It completely overwhelmed him. He couldn't stand still and face it like *B*. Probably his unconscious sent down another message to the adrenals saying: "You will simply have to let this fellow take a few counts until I lasso the complex again. Meanwhile you might give us a little more juice."

If I have given you the impression that the adrenals are the most important glands in the body I have given you a wrong one. The thyroid is as important as the adrenals, as are also the thymus, the pituitary, the ovaries and the testes. In fact, they react to and counteract each other in a most remarkable fashion. They run like a smoothly interlocking system of wheels within wheels. And when one does not function properly, either through overactivity or underactivity, it always upsets the normal functioning of the others which, in turn, will undersecrete or oversecrete, as the case requires, in order that some semblance of balance may again be restored.

During the past fifty years of the most scientifically searching and practical work on the endocrine glands, especially interesting has been the investigation of the adrenals. Noteworthy has been the correlation with the flight-fight concept at the psychological level.

The *flight-fight mechanism*, you see, actually constitutes the core of human behavior. When all is said and done, the essence of the problem is the way you and I, as individuals, respond to, and are influenced by, our environment. That is what conditions conduct.

And in this relationship between the individual on the one hand, and the world of reality on the other, lies *conflict*.

Now the individual succeeds in conquering reality; now he fails. Now he achieves his ambition, encompasses his ideals, finds and subdues the woman who gratifies his love life, makes a lot of money, allows his ego free play—all because he is winning in the fight. Now he feels discouraged and unhappy, recognizes that the goal of his ambition is still miles and miles away; his ideas have gone smash; he is still seeking, yearning, prayerfully hoping for that "one and only" through whom he will again he able to express, not only his sex, but his deepest personality cravings as well—all because life is giving him the worst of it and he is running away. Standing still is, psychologically, a running away. A definite psychological flight from reality develops an orthodox neurosis with symptoms.

Psychiatrists recognize this universally motivating flight-fight mechanism. When in flight they say you repress. Repression is the keystone of the neurotic arch.

The physiologists likewise recognize the flight-fight mechanism. The cramping and squeezing of gland energy into the musculature of the body makes for tension, like the tension of a coiled spring in a jack-in-the-box, and this compression of energy at one and the same time prevents its release.

Here we have two perfectly rational explanations to account for success and failure, for contentment and discontent, for the basic cause for achievement, for gratified love and sex and for starved love and sex. Nor is it a question of taking your choice. Both explanations dovetail and the best plan is to play both ends, not against the middle, but in conjunction with the middle.

In my own neuropsychiatric practice, fully two-thirds of all my patients receive gland therapy as well as some form of analytic procedure. Usually the primary cause is unconscious repression which, even in childhood, has affected the glandular system. The problem often resembles the one involved in the joke about which came first, the chicken or the egg. To treat either the mind or the glands alone is not enough in the out-and-out neurotic disorders. Both must receive the proper share of attention.

I touched upon the thyroid gland in relation to *B*. This gland is situated just behind and below the Adam's apple in the neck and when it is enlarged it is spoken of as a "goiter."

That the thyroid has a most significant lot to do with rousing brain activity and stimulating the intelligence, there can be no question whatsoever. Thyroid tablets are used continually in the treatment of *feeble-minded* states due to deficiency of thyroid. The way such a so-called "cretin" will change from a stunted, coarse-skinned, square-headed, wide-mouthed, ugly imbecile or idiot into a being that, in appearance and intelligence at least, has a right to claim a human classification, comes mighty close to being a miracle in an age when about the only true thing that can be said about a miracle is that there "ain't no sich animal."

Thyroid as well as other gland extracts are also given nowadays to children who are backward in school, who are shut in and asocial, who are delinquent, etc. Skill is required in such treatment and it should never be undertaken except by a medical expert in nervous and mental disorders.

It is interesting here to speculate what a few of the world's famous neurotics must have been, "glandularly" speaking.

First Napoleon, that individualist par excellence, that dynamic, ruthless genius about whose public achievements and private peccadillos more has been written than about any other human being in history. What about his adrenals and thyroid?

Being a many-sided man one might expect him not to be so simple about his gland composition. And sure enough; Napoleon was primarily a pluriglandular case—adrenals, thyroid and pituitary.

The pituitary lies in a bony, saddle-shaped bed, the *sella turcica*, at the bottom of the brain. Its anterior part, or lobe, has to do with skeletal growth; its posterior with metabolism.

Now the striking characteristic about Napoleon was, of course, his small stature (deficient secretion of the anterior lobe of the pituitary). He was domineering, irascible, supremely egotistic, indefatigable, unscrupulous—no flight but chock-full of fight (abundant adrenal activity). He tended to be corpulent and at St. Helena he got positively fat and flabby (insufficient secretion of the posterior lobe of the pituitary). He possessed a remarkable mind that functioned like a steel trap (thyroid efficiency). And then those fainting attacks of his, often spoken of as having been definite states of epileptic unconsciousness? Nowadays it is well known that pituitary disorder may be accompanied by epilepsy. Lastly, and in addition, Napoleon's sexual life. It was marked by sudden flares of desire which disappeared, if not satisfied, as quickly and unexpectedly as they had arisen. He was never in love in the sense of a lasting, idealized affection for any one particular woman (deficient gonads). Josephine had to give way when the heir that his brain demanded was not forthcoming.

What finally failed Napoleon were not his adrenals or his thyroid but his pituitary, the one weak link in his glandular chain. He was noticeably becoming fat when he made himself emperor. Impaired judgment was shown in the Russian campaign. Already the weak pituitary was beginning to unbalance the thyroid, possibly even the adrenals. We know that after Waterloo he gradually grew indolent, shut in, sulking and apathetic (subpituitary). His mental ability toward the end can be judged by that childish essay of his on suicide.

Might the story of Waterloo have ended differently had the specialists of the time known about Napoleon's pituitary insufficiency? But can you imagine him taking their advice? Can you picture him in a busy campaign stopping to take his tablet on an empty stomach three times a day?

Next I think of Oscar Wilde and of the thymus.

At birth this gland is very large and toward the end of the second year it attains its maximum growth. It then reaches, in leaflike fashion, from the root of the lungs to the base of the neck. Normally it diminishes in size after that. When puberty is reached it has almost disappeared.

What the thymus does, apparently, is to use itself up, like

a martyr, in inhibiting the development of sex structures. This seems to be necessary in the early years of life in order to avoid sex precocity. When the thymus gland does not involute in the male we find the adult's general appearance decidedly feminine. This is likewise true of his mental processes and general effeminate behavior. It is not necessary to study psychoanalysis to be convinced of that. The sexual life of these persistent thymus cases is, as might be expected, abnormal.

Had Wilde received glandular treatment and a psychoanalysis for his homosexuality in a hospital instead of being thrown into prison, the world might have saved a rare appraiser of the beautiful as well as a literary genius. But these glands of ours were not then generally recognized for what they are and Wilde was held responsible for homosexual behavior that really he could not help any more than he could the exceptional size of his skull.

I have already referred in passing to the remarkable way in which glands intercorrelate one with the other. When one is deficient another attempts, through overactivity, to compensate for the loss. Thus we see in Wilde a pituitary compensation for thymus persistence. He was tall, corpulent, and his head was large—all connected with metabolic and skeletal growth, hypersecretion of the posterior and anterior pituitary lobes respectively.

What is human nature? What is man? What is his soul? Darwin, Huxley and Herbert Spencer began the quest for an answer. They hunted in the past. Thomas Addison, Charcot, Moebius, Brown-Sequard and the rest have been concerned less with what *was* than with what *is*. Their work has been the endocrine glands. A thorough understanding and control of these glands of ours suggests almost unbelievable possibilities for the future.

Already the slow and retarded receive their thyroid; the nervous and emotionally unstable their pituitary; if the blood pressure is low and mental activity exhausts itself like a fire of straw, adrenal substance may be indicated. Emotional inadequacy and emotional instability, deception, prevarication, philandering, temper and temperament, criminality and the taking of life—each may have a little gland story of its own.

The absolute, unchallenged and irrefutable answer to the why, the wherefore and the how cannot, however, be so far off at that when these analysts and physiologists can be on speaking terms!

Be glad, therefore. As a neurotic it may be that all you need is a little glandular adjustment, the mental side then reacting sufficiently favorable to grant you your desires. And if it be a severe neurosis that holds you in its grip, glands can be made to join hands with analytic insight and speed you to victory.

Chapter XV

EVEN MEN HAVE CHANGE OF LIFE

REGARDING GLANDULAR ADJUSTMENT—OR should I say, maladjustment—one naturally thinks of middle life, say, from forty to fifty, with special emphasis placed upon that dreaded age of forty-five, the usual time for the female menopause. Now we know, however, that men also undergo a so-called change of life, in most cases at about fifty, and that they as well as women can get their nerves upset no end because of it.

To be sure, not every middle-ager develops a crisis at the climacteric. There are men who experience no difference in physical, mental or emotional tone and never realize that physiological and chemical changes are taking place within their bodies. There are women who tide over this transition year or years with little or no disturbance or discomfort of any kind. If such occur medical science is ready to lend a helping hand through the proper administration of gland hormones. Actually, it is the mental side—an unwarranted fear that from now on the individual's life is practically finished—that drives a considerable number of men as well as women into a state of alarm.

There was the case of Mr. J. At fifty he was a top-flight executive of a large manufacturing concern, earning $50,000 a year and generally considered one of the most intelligent and successful men in the business. So well was he thought of that during the Second World War the government frequently called him in for consultation. His impressive figure, six feet tall and muscular, matched his forceful personality. He was specially known for the confidence he inspired and for the sureness with which he handled men.

But this is what his wife said of him: "Something's come over Ted lately that I cannot understand. He complains of headaches, of occasional dizziness and he doesn't sleep well," she said. "Whereas formerly he always liked to see the children and fuss over our two granddaughters, he now avoids them and is irritable when they are around. He is impatient with me, too, and I am told that he is irritable at the office and gets into loud arguments. What particularly alarmed me was his saying last night that for two pins he'd put an end to it all. After that I felt it was high time he consulted a psychiatrist."

Actually, however, there was nothing to be alarmed about. J's neurotic manifestations were merely those characteristic of a change of life. A few weeks of endocrine therapy, plus several psychoanalytic talks, straightened him out and made him over, to use his own words, "as good as new."

Many other symptoms besides those that assailed J may attend the male climacteric. Tension is a common symptom, likewise depression and emotional instability that may lead to tearfulness and spells of weeping. Such persons tire readily and complain of not being able to concentrate. Memory can be poor, especially as regards recent events and the names of persons well known to them. Feelings of anxiety, depression, despair and a sense of impending danger may be marked. A loss of interest in work, friends and family is the rule. These are avoided and the patient prefers being alone, refusing to go out socially or to visit the theater or movies. All sorts of trifling things annoy and worry him. Inferiority ideas develop. He thinks he will lose his job because he is not efficient any more. He talks of growing old and being useless. Whereas formerly active and ambitious, such a man now becomes indolent and indifferent. And, of course, secretly he keeps worrying about losing his manhood because he notes a decline or loss of potency.

On the physical side hot flushes may be the rule as in the case of women. Numbness of hands and feet, also tingling sensations in the extremities, and pains here and there, may be experienced. Palpitation, shortness of breath and fear of a physical illness, such as cancer, heart disease or a stroke, are encountered.

There may be other manifestations, as well, that give rise to alarm. These concern philandering ideas and tendencies.

Many a man has got himself into difficulties when he found his sex desires decreasing and became convinced that what he needed was the stimulus of strange and younger women. Such wayward interests tend, of course, to be carried to excess, and the added strain on glandular structures in the process of natural evolution is to weaken them all the more.

Tolerance and understanding, even forgiveness, are required at such a crucial time in a man's life. Although it is particularly hard on a wife, what such a person needs is neither a scolding nor threats. He should be made to realize, rather, that no one has lost faith in him, either in his working ability, his love for his family or in his moral stamina. The patient's philandering tendencies can and should be shunted back as quickly as possible into some form of ego build-up that will rout his growing inferiority convictions.

Then, of course, medical treatment also is indicated. The administration of testosterone in one form or another is the preferred way of giving the body what it is being depleted of too rapidly. In a few weeks or months—cases vary—this sex hormone usually accomplishes wonders. As the endocrine structure is aided and tided over, as it were, and a new equilibrium between the glands concerned is established, symptoms disappear, emotional equilibrium is restored, mental powers reappear and physical well-being, even in the sexual sphere, is experienced.

Impotence, as such, can also be purely psychic and have no reference whatever to the crucial climacteric years of the male, say, between forty-five and fifty-five, with exceptions as early as thirty-five and as late as past sixty. Indeed, I have met with many cases of such sexual impotence in youths of twenty-five and younger.

These latter cases are purely neurotic in origin and usually the result of some guilt-punishment mechanism that is unconscious. When it occurs in married men whose sex life has been satisfactory heretofore, the cause may be some conscious or unconscious antagonism to the wife which is not recognized because it is disguised.

Psychic impotence is seldom if ever benefited by gland treatment. A thoroughgoing psychoanalysis is always indicated. As regards what might be called neurotic manifestations in an apparently nonneurotic male suffering from change of life, analysis also is desirable although in a less intensive way.

It has been estimated that 95 per cent of all men pass

through a change of life without being upset in any way, or if they are it is so mild in character that they take it in their stride without comment or complaint. The figures are exactly the reverse of the female. Ninety-five per cent of all women are affected nervously to greater or lesser degree as their menstrual periods become less marked and irregular and finally disappear. Only 5 per cent note no special changes in their physical or emotional reactions as such.

Yet women need not worry at all. For them estrogen works as effectively as testosterone does for men. Unfortunately, when a woman undergoes the menopause her physical appearance changes, and this causes her more unhappy moments than all the physical and emotional symptoms, shown by men as well, put together. When her skin tends to grow flabby, increased weight is revealed at the wrong places and wrinkles show on her face and neck, when her hair thins and a faint suggestion of a mustache appears, then it is that neurotic symptoms of almost any variety can spring into being.

Indeed, many women don't wait to develop a case of nerves until the menopause is reached. They start a few years earlier before the "dreaded age of forty" arrives. Indeed, this forty-phobia may appear in the early thirties.

As if an atomic bomb were threatening, women then begin to look frightened when their age is questioned, their visits to the beauty parlor become more and more frequent, cosmetics deplete their purses more and more completely. A certain conviction of utter frustration and hopelessness seems to mount as that awful fortieth birthday draws nearer and nearer. I have seen otherwise happy women become miserable and bitter. Devastating ideas of inferiority and uselessness may become an obsession.

Luckily, not all women go neurotic that way. Many accept the inevitable forties with resignation and try to compensate by developing new interests and a new outlook on life. By far and large, however, the forties present a most favorable soil for the sprouting of hitherto dormant neurotic tendencies or for the precipitation of an actual and distressing neurosis.

Behind all this fear, and motivating it since girlhood, is the instinctive urge of every woman to love and be loved.

What the average woman craves above all else is neither social position, artistic achievement, fame, money, clothes, jewels, furs, a career or her picture in the magazines. What she wants is *love*. And what she dreads is the possibility, when in the forties, that she will lose love.

The forty-phobia is, nevertheless, purely a mirage. As the woman catches up with her apprehensions, so to speak, and finds herself safely past forty and getting along well in spite of it, her fear gradually disappears as does mist before the sun.

Tradition—a false and pernicious one at that—is largely responsible for women believing that, since the reproductive period ends at the menopause, the poor, worn-out, old lady from now on should sit by the fire and knit. A similar foolish notion exists regarding her sex life. As a matter of fact, sex can be as important, if not more important, to a woman after the climacteric than before. Freed from the danger and fear of pregnancy many a woman enjoys her physical relationships as never before. Frigidity, too—practically always a mental affair—may likewise disappear automatically.

What a woman should try particularly to do as middle life

approaches is stress and express her individuality. The list of women who did just that, who refused to be alarmed or be by-passed by life and old-fashioned notions, and who started a brand-new career is, indeed, a long one.

Mrs. Hortense Odlum's most important job was that of wife and mother. But children grow up and the time arrives when life calls for readjustment. For Mrs. Odlum another career, demanding but immensely satisfying, began. As head of the fashionable Bonwit Teller store on New York's Fifth Avenue, she became known as one of the most brilliant merchandising executives in the country. Mrs. Emily Post had years of gracious living behind her as well as fame as a hostess among her friends before she wrote the book that has made her name synonymous with etiquette. Mary Margaret McBride carved out a career as a newspaper writer until the bottom dropped out of it with the depression. Undaunted, but with fear and trembling, she started over again in radio. Few stars of the networks can boast of as vast and enthusiastic an audience of women fans as she. Mme. Curie still was proving secrets of radioactivity (precursor of the atom bomb) when she was well along into advanced years that would have spelled old age to most of us.

At forty you possess an outlook on life that is valuable and should be put to practical use. Social work, politics, women's clubs with a serious sociological or charitable purpose are all open to you. Life still holds for you endless possibilities if only you will bestir yourself to find them. Find your own niche in the world and fill it with honor.

During middle life, too, women gradually find themselves quieting down in regard to their nervous constitution. They develop more poise and emotional stability. Whether she has been married or not, has had children or not, has failed or not according to her own thinking, this turning point in life is exactly the time for a woman to make a new and fresh start.

Be *yourself!* Don't imitate or try to fit yourself into the pattern of others. Stop worrying about what other people think. Free yourself from this devastating fixation left over from childhood. Be mature and stand on your own two feet. Don't try to dress and behave as though you were an adolescent. Be original in your clothes. Try to make them enhance and etch your personality.

Last, but not least, that's the way to avoid becoming neurotic.

Chapter XVI

HOW NEUROTIC ARE YOU ANYWAY? TRY THIS TEST

THERE ARE THOSE WHO BELIEVE THEY ARE not neurotic when actually they are; there are those, also, who are not so neurotic as they think they are.

But why not have "the truth, the whole truth and nothing but the truth"? Take the time to do the following test and check up on your nerves. It will remove much of the doubt and confusion you have about yourself. It will be an illuminating as well as refreshing experience.

Don't, however, allow this test to frighten you. After all, while some possess the knack of evaluating their own handicaps, others find such self-analysis difficult. If you will consider this test as a general guide only, you will approach it with the best point of view. It should make you glad to discover that others have symptoms you do not possess.

A Test to Check Up on Your Nerves

Read These Directions Carefully

1. First read the 50 questions over carefully, at least once, to get a general idea of the subject matter.
2. In doing this, note that most of the questions really consist of two questions separated by or. That is why there are two "yes" columns at the right.
3. If, therefore, you answer the first part of such a double question in the affirmative, place a check in the first "Yes" column; if only the second, then a check should be placed in the second column. And, of course, if your answer is an affirmative one for both parts of the question, then two checks will appear opposite the question.

4. A few questions, you will note further, consist of one question alone. Such, for example, is 11, which inquires whether you are *self-conscious*. Should you be suffering from this complaint *two* checks should be placed opposite the question. In other words, either you are self-conscious or you *are not*. If you are, it counts more heavily in making an analysis of yourself than if, for instance, you are only *afraid to meet people*, the second part of Question 1.
5. It must be remembered that even marked neurotic symptoms may have their normal and average counterparts, therefore do not score yourself a Yes unless your trait is really definite, marked and at least somewhat bothersome. Everybody is more or less *sensitive*, for instance (first part of Question 1) but such average amount of sensitiveness is something quite different from being *oversensitive*.
6. It cannot be emphasized too strongly, on the other hand, that the general tendency is to make excuses for oneself—to "let oneself down easy"—rather than to overstate one's faults; although people do exist who, just because they are neurotic, delight in finding fault with themselves.
7. After you have finished scoring yourself, add up all the check marks in both "Yes" columns and subtract from 100. The remainder will reveal to you how nearly normal—it would be better to say *average*—you are, and in terms of per cent.
8. It is not possible for anyone to score 100 per cent. Absolute normality does not exist. If you have 15 checks or less, making you 85 per cent normal or better, I am afraid this book roused in you merely an academic interest. A score of 70 to 85 checks would tend to indicate that you may place yourself in the neurotic class, which I hope, by now, you consider a privilege. A person who scores more than 85 checks is probably suffering from a severe neurosis.

How Neurotic Are You Anyway? Try This Test

A Test to Check Up on Your Nerves

Score Box

	Yes	Yes
1. Are you OVERSENSITIVE *or* AFRAID to MEET PEOPLE?		
2. Do you AVOID SOCIAL CONTACTS *or* REMAIN too much BY YOURSELF?		
3. Do you indulge in SELF-PITY *or* tend to PAMPER YOURSELF?		
4. Are you given to SELF-ACCUSATION *or* to feelings of GUILT?		
5. Are you quick to make EXCUSES for yourself *or* DEFEND YOURSELF before others?		
6. Are you OVERCONSCIENTIOUS to the point where it annoys you?		
7. Do you feel REPRESSED *or* feel that you could do CREATIVE WORK?		
8. Any feelings of ANXIETY *or* IMPENDING DANGER without knowing why?		
9. Are you given to WORRY WITHOUT JUSTIFICATION *or* are you forever concerned about WHAT PEOPLE THINK?		
10. Are you convinced, but without justification, that you are either INFERIOR *or* SUPERIOR to others?		
11. Do you suffer from SELF-CONSCIOUSNESS?		
12. Are you assailed by the habit of DOUBT, not knowing what is best to do *or* are you unusually SUGGESTIBLE		
13. Are you JEALOUS *or* SUSPICIOUS of others?		
14. Are you extremely CRITICAL of others *or* DIFFICULT TO PLEASE?		
15. Are you unable to MAKE *or* HOLD FRIENDS?		
16. Do you EXAGGERATE trifles *or* unduly MINIMIZE important things?		
17. Are you either DEPRESSED *or* unduly OPTIMISTIC without cause?		
18. Are you continually DISSATISFIED *or* upset by MENTAL CONFLICTS?		
19. Do you PREFER the society of the SAME SEX *or* DISLIKE THE OPPOSITE SEX?		

A TEST TO CHECK UP ON YOUR NERVES.—(*Continued*)

	Score Box	
	Yes	Yes
20. Are you "HEART-HUNGRY" *or* do your SEX DESIRES TANTALIZE?		
21. Do you DISLIKE CHILDREN *or* feel ANTAGONISTIC toward MARRIAGE?		
22. Do you DAYDREAM a great deal *or* do you FAIL TO TRY to make your ambitions come true?		
23. Have you LOST INTEREST IN CURRENT EVENTS *or* do you feel DISGUSTED WITH THE WORLD?		
24. Do you tend to be RADICAL just to be different *or* are you stubbornly CONSERVATIVE?		
25. Have you become generally FAULT-FINDING *or* CYNICAL?		
26. Have you LOST AMBITION *or* do you feel your LIFE has been a FAILURE?		
27. Do you LACK SELF-CONFIDENCE *or* feel you would like to be A CHILD AGAIN?		
28. Do you often feel that PEOPLE *or* YOUR SURROUNDINGS ARE UNREAL?		
29. Are you UNABLE TO HOLD ANY JOB FOR LONG?		
30. Are you exceptionally ORDERLY *or* unusually DISORDERLY?		
31. Are you OVERCAREFUL in DRESSING *or* do you spend an excessive amount of TIME BEFORE THE MIRROR?		
32. Do you consider yourself a PHYSICAL COWARD *or* do you LIE even when it is not necessary?		
33. Are you SUPERSTITIOUS *or* do you adhere to any CULT of any kind?		
34. Is the influence of a PARENT *or* ANY RELATIVE unusually strong?		
35. Do you frequently make ERRORS *or* do things you CONSIDER FOOLISH?		
36. Any COMPULSIONS such as looking into closets, under the bed, satisfying yourself several times that the door is locked, the gas off, etc., *or* are you unable to overcome any BAD HABITS, such as excessive use of tobacco, alcohol, etc.?		

A TEST TO CHECK UP ON YOUR NERVES.—(*Continued*)

Score Box	Yes	Yes
37. Have you a haunting DREAD OF DEATH?		
38. Have you a passion for COLLECTING THINGS *or* do you QUICKLY TIRE and GET RID of your belongings?		
39. Do you FEAR THE DARK or any of the FORCES OF NATURE *or* suffer a DREAD OF INSANITY?		
40. Do you think about committing SUICIDE *or* entertain other MORBID IDEAS?		
41. Do you feel UNCOMFORTABLE IN CLOSED PLACES such as elevators, subways, etc., *or* when traversing OPEN SPACES such as fields, plazas, etc.?		
42. Do you DISLIKE HIGH PLACES such as mountains, tall buildings, etc., *or* do you have an IMPULSE to jump off?		
43. Any unreasonable FEAR OF GERMS *or* has CLEANLINESS become an OBSESSION?		
44. Are you IRRITABLE *or* given to TEMPER TANTRUMS?		
45. Is your CONCENTRATION *or* MEMORY poor?		
46. Are you easily FATIGUED *or* do you feel you must ALWAYS "BE ON THE GO?"		
47. Do you find it DIFFICULT to RELAX *or* do you suffer from INSOMNIA?		
48. Do you have frequent HEADACHES *or* are you generally UNSTABLE EMOTIONALLY?		
49. Do you have DISTURBING DREAMS *or* do you tend to OVERSLEEP?		
50. Have you PHYSICAL SYMPTOMS that doctors claim are IMAGINARY?		

Totals (add both columns)..................

Chapter XVII

BEING NEUROTIC, SHOULD YOU MARRY?

A YOUNG WOMAN WAS USHERED INTO MY consulting room one day, the picture of dejection and despair. From the look of her dull, red eyes it was evident that she had been weeping as well as suffering from loss of sleep. Taking the proffered chair at my desk she kept pulling at her handkerchief and with lowered head fixed her gaze on the floor.

"Please tell me what is distressing you so," I asked with as much encouragement as possible. "Just talking it out should help, you know."

For a few seconds she neither moved nor replied when suddenly, as though making a supreme effort, she turned and whispered hoarsely: "The boy I was going to marry has been sent home a mental case." Then she broke down and sobbed as though her heart would break.

Thousands of women—wives, mothers and sweethearts—have been shocked like that during the last war. As in the case of the girl just cited, many of the folks at home were not only astonished but actually stunned when something like this happened. Because of nerves, strong, virile and capable men were classified as 4-F by their local draft boards, others were discharged while in training and still others "broke down" and were returned as unfit for military duty. Few suspected that any maladjustment of any kind existed, and to be placed in the 4-F category for a "mental" reason carried with it, in their opinion, a kind of stigma that, somehow, vaguely reflected upon the other members of the family. All of which, of course, was absurd.

What had disturbed the young woman mentioned above was, to be sure, the fear that marriage with her ex-soldier friend was out of the question, which also proved to be ridiculous. For this young man was not a mental case at all—this designation being used correctly only when applying to a psychosis. His diagnosis upon discharge was psychoneurosis.

The term *psychoneurosis* is an old one that, for the most part, has been discarded. It means the same thing as *neurosis.* Psychoneurosis and neurosis, therefore, are interchangeable terms.

At the various induction centers 1,825,000 out of 4,650,000 men were rejected because of a personality maladjustment. There were 300,000 discharged from the Army for neuropsychiatric reasons. The total percentage of the two groups reaches the astounding figure of 43. In the Navy, 37,100 men were discharged with the diagnosis "psychoneurosis" from Jan. 1, 1942, through June, 1945. To believe that these hundreds of thousands of men taken from civilian life, where the vast majority held jobs, supported themselves and often families in addition and otherwise conducted themselves in an intelligent and adequate manner could or should, by far and large, be looked upon as in any way deficient, inferior, unbalanced or otherwise unfit, is preposterous. I know personally of a score or more of highly intelligent, unusually efficient men who were classified by the Army as neurotic. Among these are business and professional men of outstanding ability who draw large salaries and are most respected in the communities in which they live. Indeed, it is a well-known fact that many of the high officials in Washington, who actually conducted the war, were neurotic themselves!

Even members of Congress did not escape the 4-F classification. It was an amusing sidelight on psychoneurotic labeling to read that these officials resented it. They were inclined to believe that such a psychoneurotic designation placed them in a false position before the public. People might think they were incompetent for their jobs!

In a paper read before the American Psychiatric Association in May, 1944, Lieut. Col. Malcolm J. Farrell and Capt. John W. Appel of the Army Medical Corps exploded the popular myth that only weaklings develop psychiatric upsets. "In one campaign," the report stated, "the incidence of psychiatric cases was uniformly higher among veteran combat troops than among fresh, green troops. Months of intensive combat had weeded out all the weaklings. The men who remained had proved the toughness of their underlying personality structure by their mere survival. Yet fatigue and other factors produced more 'psychoneurotics' among this group than among fresh, untried troops. In short, it became evident that anybody could develop a psychoneurosis under certain circumstances."

In other words, everybody has a breaking point.

Imagine what would happen if Joseph Pulitzer, famous founder of the *New York World*, had appeared for a selective service examination. The clink of a stethoscope, the clank of a weight on a scale balance, would probably have driven him frantic, for he was so incredibly sensitive to sound that the rasp of a fork on a dinner plate was enough to bring down a tirade upon the offender. Yet Pulitzer is an immortal name in American journalism.

John Bunyan was a neurotic who saw strange visions—but we still read *Pilgrim's Progress*. Thomas De Quincey was an opium addict; William Seabury presented an enthralling personal picture of alcohol addiction in his book *Asylum*; Leo Tolstoy, a titan of literature, was beset with powerful obsessions and compulsions that were surely psychoneurotic.

Yes, among the most brilliant names of history you'll encounter neurotic after neurotic who certainly would never have got beyond the psychiatric screening test of a military board.

The same question may be raised regarding a host of other famous men and women already mentioned in this book. The greatest thinkers and doers in all walks of life: musicians, writers, actors, inventors, sculptors, painters, astronomers, research workers and professors of all kinds, as well as the builders of big business, are either neurotic or actually suffer from neurosis. May I emphasize again that neurotics are, fundamentally, superior people whether or not they have found themselves, whether or not they are still repressed and in conflict with themselves. Because of this inherent, dynamic force that can be released, they should be glad.

No woman need fear marrying a neurotic nor should any man hesitate about going to the altar with a neurotic woman.

A husband who is neurotic possesses a high degree of sensitivity that may make him a bit touchy, that may make his feelings easily hurt. He may likewise require a great deal of attention, even to the extent of wanting to be babied. He will probably be critical and faultfinding but with the idea of having as perfect and as well-run a home as possible. However, since a neurotic possesses an abundance of feeling, his capacity for love, loyalty and consideration for his partner is large. In short, a neurotic has the makings for an exceptionally fine husband.

The same may be said of a neurotic wife. Although her emotional ups and downs may be trying at times and she probably will demand repeated proof that she is truly loved, life with her will, at least, never be humdrum.

Three tendencies must, however, be controlled. These are *emotional immaturity*, *overpossessiveness* and *sexual incompatibility.*[1]

Neurotics, being more or less autoerotic and not yet having rid themselves of their emotional puppy wool, sometimes find it difficult to transfer affection, in the spirit of true surrender, to members of the opposite sex. They are unwilling to make advances, preferring to be courted themselves. This applies to men as well as to women. A parent fixation may, of course, be the important causative factor involved. No person can hope to make a go of marriage if he or she has not yet emancipated himself sufficiently from parental influence or domination.

Overpossessiveness is a criticism frequently encountered in cases of marital incompatibility. One charges the other as wanting to usurp all the time and attention available. "I'm watched and supervised all day long, even while at work. I feel as if I'm in a prison with no sense of freedom," complains a husband. A wife may cry: "Since our marriage, I can't call my soul my own. My life is worse than that of a slave. He

[1] Chap. XI might be reviewed here with profit.

wants me to wait on him and respond to his beck and call whenever it suits his fancy." Such unhappy ones must learn to realize that, in the last analysis, it is love that is motivating such possessive desires. A toning down is indicated here. Separate vacations once or twice a year, friends, hobbies and amusements can do wonders.

When sexual incompatibility is encountered from whatever cause and it cannot be straightened out through the reading of popular books on the subject, a visit should be made to a competent psychiatrist.

Nor is there any reason why two people with neurotic tendencies should not marry. Tempers may flash and flare now and again, and, as one such couple described their relationship, "there's never a dull moment"; nevertheless, I have known dozens and dozens of such marriages that were far happier than the average. Like understands like.

I would, however, caution a woman against marrying a man who suffers from a well-defined neurosis in contrast to his being merely neurotic. The same would apply to a man contemplating marriage with such a woman. Marked fears, compulsions, hypochondriacal ideas and asthenia (pronounced physical weakness but on an emotional basis) make a poor and faulty foundation for the building of a home and happiness. What such individuals should do is to be cured first—then marry. The experience of having battled a neurosis and then of having been cured by means of a thoroughgoing psychoanalysis should make of such individuals the very best of marital partners.

Hereditary factors do not, of course, exist. You do not transmit your neurosis, nor even a tendency toward it, to your children. Your neurotic disposition and attitude can, however, set a favorable groundwork for neurotic development in your child. It is the neurotic family environment in childhood as well as the child's reaction to it that counts.

Repression in childhood can, of course, produce neurosis. On the other hand, no child can or should be allowed to grow up an untrained savage who is unmindful of the rights of others. Perhaps the best yardstick to follow is this: "Train your child in such a way as to avoid guilt and inferiority as much as possible."

Coerce him and, if necessary, punish him. Do it always, however, with understanding, never in anger, and try always to make him understand why you do what you do. Be fair, too, and don't withhold praise. Remember that he has a sensitive ego that should not be hurt too much. Bestow your love, don't withhold it, but be careful not to overdo such affection. See to it that your child believes he is wanted, that he belongs and that he feels secure and unafraid within the family circle.

Regarding sex education, don't keep your child "innocent" too long no matter how appealing that may seem. Don't curb his sex curiosity but answer his questions frankly and in a way that he can understand at his age. Many books can be secured on sex training for children of various ages.

And, particularly, don't be shocked or look dismayed if you discover onanism to have become a habit. Talk it out or seek advice elsewhere as how best to meet this situation. Usually a boy or girl will benefit by a visit to the family doctor. But whatever you do, don't lie to him or her about anything sexual. You may want to wait until the child is older before becoming too specific. Then tell him so. It is no longer considered cute to have children believe the stork or other similar fable when their companions are giving these the lie. Lastly, never frighten him with nonsensical stories about masturbation leading to insanity or other mental or physical injury.

Thousands of returning veterans want to marry, and a considerable proportion of these either are neurotic or they are oppressed by a neurosis. What I have just written about neurotics and marriage applies to them as well.

In my opinion it is hazardous for any ex-service man to rush into marriage irrespective of his neurotic status. To be sure, absence makes the heart grow fonder, and the young men, after what they have endured in the way of loneliness and hardship, are eager for affection, female companionship and a home. A cooling-off period as regards the emotions after their return is nevertheless desirable. It takes time to readjust oneself to civilian ways and modes of thinking. In addition, there is always that matter of a job or of more schooling.

Women should keep such facts in mind and never bring pressure to bear where marriage with a recent veteran is concerned. It is better to curb one's desires, hopes and enthusiasm and wait for the time when the boy friend really is ready. The chances for a lasting union are infinitely better that way.

Chapter XVIII

LEARN HOW TO CONTROL YOUR FUTURE

WHEN YOU WERE A CHILD YOU WERE UNable to control your environment. Until about the age of five your reasoning, judgment, powers of comparison and the rest of your intellectual faculties were scarcely functioning. For years after that, even, your parents, your teachers, your surroundings, were dominating factors in shaping your thoughts and feelings, in establishing the character of your unconscious mind. You had little, if anything, to do with your repressions and complexes, with your maladjustments and symptoms.

Now, however, it is different! You are an adult. You may still be influenced overmuch by your emotional make-up laid down in the past. Your intellect, nevertheless, no matter how much it may be undermined by unconscious mechanisms, is mature; your conscious mind likewise possesses the independence of maturity to greater or lesser degree. You now can change the present and plan ahead. What is generally recognized as *will power* is at your service.

In other words—and aside from overcoming your neurosis, mild or severe—*you can learn how to control your future!*

What you must specially guard against, what you must prepare for, is not so much what is likely to take place as what is *unlikely* to occur. It makes no difference who you are, what you are, what you have been or what you hope to be, the unexpected may happen and change everything. It is the *unexpected,* not our own preparation for the future, that so often shapes our lives.

Primo Carnera was a carpenter and content to remain so for the rest of his days. But chance led him into a circus where the manager, impressed by his giant frame, offered him the job of strong man in the side show. Weeks later, also by chance, a sports promoter happened to witness his feats of strength and persuaded him to take on Leon Sebillo, an experienced 200-pound boxer. Carnera knocked out his adversary in the very first round. The unexpected happened for the third time! The carpenter became a professional pugilist.

If Lew Fields had not been amused at the way Vernon Castle draped his long, spindle legs around himself when he happened to meet him at a stag party in New York, there probably never would have been a stage career for Castle nor would ballroom dancing have become the vogue he made it.

I am acquainted with a woman whose husband died suddenly of a heart attack, when she was forty-six years old. With consternation she learned that he had left her without a cent. After repeated failure to secure any kind of employment whatsoever, and with starvation imminent, she decided finally to turn on the gas and end it all. She determined, however, not to leave this world without an explanation, without attempting to justify herself. But as she was finishing her "apologia," the bell rang and a newspaper friend stood at the door. That story turned out to be such a revealing human document that the friend was able to have it published. Within a few months the would-be suicide was writing for the "pulps," still wondering how it all happened.

Learn How to Control Your Future

One never can tell! *Chance* plays such a tremendously important role in our lives. Trace your own past and you will find more than one instance to corroborate this. So many are there likely to be, in fact, that you may wonder whether any of them could possibly have been controlled in advance. The life that is entirely uneventful, where the unexpected never happens, is rare indeed. The long arm of circumstance frequently may single us out to alter the course of our careers, to influence our success, to sway our love relationships and to modify the state of our happiness. In fact, when the unexpected happens other things happen as well. Changes result, either for better or for worse. The effect of the unexpected, because it is usually sudden, sharp and dramatic, is telling.

It is when the unexpected carries *bad* news, however, that devastating troubles usually start. Think how you would feel if, quite out of a clear sky, you lost your job or your savings, or you were seriously injured or laid low with a chronic disease? Such contemplation is not pleasant, I know. Nor is the fact that some day we die—an event for which we also should prepare.

Although bad news and unexpected disaster are admittedly upsetting, one might think that *good* news surely could produce no harm. Strangely enough, unexpected happiness can tear up the emotions worse than sorrow. That's because we never are taken as much by surprise when the unexpected spells sadness as when it spells gladness. Most of us, you see, already have suffered aplenty and we are more or less used to it. The expression to "die of joy" is really no mere figure of speech. To surprise old people, for example, is dangerous, especially if it carries pleasure. The same holds true for the chronically ill, for those with heart trouble and for those whose nervous system is high-strung and unstable.

But how, you may ask, can the future be controlled? How can the unexpected be prepared for when we must, by the very nature of the definition of the unexpected character of the future, remain ignorant of how and when the blow will fall? Can we protect ourselves against the onslaughts of the unexpected before it happens? Can we make ourselves more resistive? Can we fortify ourselves against the shock? Can the evil effects of the unexpected be sidetracked or halted?

Thanks to modern psychology there is an answer for each of these questions and it is a reassuring, hopeful and stimulating answer. Specifically this psychology deals with the *emotions*. Indeed, when it comes to the conquering of a serious problem brought about by the occurrence of the unexpected, the intellectual side of our brain as such offers precious little help.

Many a business executive has failed in putting through an important transaction for no other reason than that he quarreled with his wife at breakfast. Students who know their subjects frequently fail in examinations because of fear. Stage fright is the besetting sin of the actor. "I was too nervous" is a common excuse among women. In all such cases the mental faculties are as sound anatomically as ever. But they do not function as well as they should because emotion undermines their efficiency.

That is exactly what takes place in the human being when the unexpected lays him low. The possession of a trained mind may heighten the wall of personal fortification. Everybody, however, has a "breaking point." How to avoid such a break of morale, possibly a nervous collapse—how to escape being overwhelmed, is the problem.

I stated that you actually can protect yourself against the unexpected before it happens. You really can make yourself resistive to most eventualities the future may carry. Especially should those that commonly occur be prepared for; these being illness, injury, loss of a faculty, paralysis, death of a beloved one, loss of job or fortune, disappointment in love. Nor is deep psychological study required. All that is necessary is a little thought and practice. In fact, in preparing yourself for the unexpected you really "kill two birds with one stone"; in making yourself resistive to chance, in fortifying yourself against a sudden attack upon your deepest and most sacred emotions, you are at one and the same time expanding and enriching your life.

Specifically make yourself *resistive* by avoiding a single goal. In other words, never concentrate on one objective to the neglect of other interests.

For instance, there was a girl, an only child and orphaned, who determined long before marriage that she would make of herself a model wife and mother. In college she chose for her elective subjects cooking, home economics and care of babies. After graduation she went so far as to work six months in a day nursery and six months as a probationary nurse. Nor did she experience any difficulty having suitors. She married, deeply in love, at twenty-three.

The unexpected that the future held for this young woman descended in her case as early as the honeymoon in France and brought to naught all her dreams. She learned from hospital records in Paris that her own father had died in that city of a disease known as haemophilia when she was six. In this disorder the "bleeder" does not transmit his condition to his daughters directly but the daughters, who are never themselves affected, transmit the haemophilia to their own sons. Naturally, children for her were out of the question. The long arm of circumstance, amazingly long in this case, shocked her so that she had to spend the rest of her honeymoon in a sanitarium.

Although I am not decrying the advantages of perfection in any one particular field of endeavor, I have seen it happen again and again that, when some dreadful disaster befell a cherished ambition, the individual literally went to pieces. That was true when a portrait painter of my acquaintance suffered a paralytic stroke after which he could not handle a brush for months, and during his convalescence losing all interest in his work. Only after some years of effort was an adjustment worked out and he became an art critic for a magazine. Had painting not been his "life and soul," as he once boastingly declared before a blood vessel burst in his brain, his interests undoubtedly would have been wider and he would have been able to "find himself" much sooner and with fewer heartaches.

As regards one's work, it is a wise plan to develop a hobby different from one's regular job. Not only is such a hobby refreshing to tired nerves but in an emergency, when regular work must be dispensed with, it can be used as a substitute, possibly even a lucrative one. The fostering of creative occupations is especially valuable here—writing, painting, sculpture, music, metalwork and other handicrafts. Bob Davis, one of the best known of magazine editors, developed portrait photography as a hobby while still the head of the Munsey publications. In the beginning he took photographs of well-known people in his office. After the magazines were discontinued he developed this hobby until his photographs of celebrities the world over now are famous and eagerly sought.

Particularly should we widen our interests where the love life is concerned. Here, to be sure, I am not advocating philandering for men or sex looseness on the part of women. I wish to emphasize, however, that men and women both make the greatest mistake when, after marriage or a formal engagement, they cut themselves off entirely from their friends. Nothing is worse than when the unexpected robs a woman of her husband in death, or vice versa, especially when they have been happily married for years. Another terrific blow to wife or husband is the sudden discovery that the other has been "cheating." Old friends of both sexes then are a great comfort as well as valuable objects toward whom to turn the tide of affection and love. The same applies regarding children. Married folks should have children and always more than one. Indeed, adopted children are better than none. Then, should the unexpected stalk ghostlike into the home, the love that is distributed among many instead of being concentrated upon one becomes a cushioned bulwark that prevents the victim from being swept out into the sea.

Fortify yourself also against the emotional shock of the unexpected by reading literature and seeing plays and movies that actually depend for interest upon the unexpected. Mystery and detective stories are excellent. Shock yourself often in a vicarious manner and you won't be so shocked when the unexpected of a frightening or even harrowing nature occurs in real life. For the time being it may not make you glad but you surely will be glad later.

If you knew that some day you would be in a shipwreck the common-sense thing to do would be to harden yourself as much as possible with adventures, actual or substitute, that would simulate an actual case. Experience would then find your emotions stabilized because already they would have been trained to that particular variety of excitement.

In Brittany, in the Basque country and other places where the population lives by fishing which is dangerous, the boys are taken out in the boats by their fathers while still in their teens, and the more frightened they are the better the oldsters like it. During both World Wars an attempt was always made to accustom men to the sound of heavy firing before they were sent to the front lines. Sham battles, also military and naval maneuvers generally, serve this purpose in addition to teaching the men how to shoot. Football practice, training for boxing and wrestling, in fact all athletic preparation, has the same psychology behind it—a hardening of the individual against the unexpected which should, after all, be expected.

Despite the most careful preparation to control one's future, it is still possible that the unexpected may be of a nature that was not even remotely anticipated. It is therefore a fair question to ask whether the evil effects of the unexpected can be sidetracked and halted.

It is in this very field that some of the most marvelous adjustments have been made. Even permanent disability has been turned into an asset. The very handicap that the unexpected handed the victim has been used by him to his own particular advantage, to make himself glad. As if to make amends to the unfortunate for his loss, nerve energy often stimulates the mind as never before and the individual excels signally for the very fact that the unexpected did occur. It is held by critics that Milton would not have been able to turn out his masterpiece *Paradise Lost* had he not been blind. One would expect deafness to be an insurmountable obstacle to a musician, yet Beethoven was handicapped that way and his greatest works were done when the deafness was complete.

The definite relationship that exists between chronic incapacity—in other words, the advent of the unexpected extending over a long period—and genius is most interesting. One wonders if the very fact of illness is not often directly responsible for greatness.[1] Indeed, the list of such persons who suffered poor health is extremely long.

Arkwright,[2] the inventor of the spinning jenny, as well as James Watt, the inventor of the steam engine, suffered wretched health. Of Voltaire and also of Rousseau it has been said that they were "born dying." After twenty-four Carlyle was an invalid, complaining that "a rat is continually gnawing at the pit of my stomach." The saints, of course, often ascribed their turning to God to the unexpected, especially when the unexpected took the form of severe illness. For example, Loyola was converted when a cannonball, at the siege of Pamplona, shattered one leg; St. Francis of Assisi was dissipated until he fell ill; St. Theresa of Jesus' accomplishments were most remarkable when she was ill and old. Coleridge first took opium by chance in a patent medicine. Julius

[1] See Chap. XX, on overcompensation.

[2] Statistical material in this paragraph taken from *The Privilege of Pain* by Mrs. Leo Everett, and by permission of Bruce Humphries, Inc., Boston, copyright owners.

Caesar and Alexander the Great suffered repeated attacks of nerves. Scores were neurotics. When Wolfe, at thirty-two, started his campaign for the conquering of Quebec, he was tortured by a chronic internal disease. Elizabeth Barrett Browning was always in delicate health. Charles Lamb and his sister had repeated attacks of insanity. Heinrich Heine struggled all his life on a "mattress grave." Darwin once said: "If I had not been so great an invalid, I should not have done nearly so much work as I have accomplished." Indeed, in reviewing the literature it would seem that about the only two outstanding geniuses who enjoyed robust health were Leonardo da Vinci and Goethe.

Unusually striking is the fact that so many individuals whose genius depends upon the productivity of their imagination suffered with tuberculosis. Robert Louis Stevenson is a classical example. Aubrey Beardsley, famous for his extraordinary black and white drawings, was a sufferer who died from the disease at twenty-six. Keats was a consumptive and there can be no question but that his genius flowered in direct proportion to the spread of his lung lesions.

When the unexpected happens another way to make it a blessing in disguise is to see whether or not it can be turned into financial profit. Certainly some persons have deliberately made money out of their afflictions. It is said that Garbo suffers from anemia. Is this the reason for her melancholy voice, her peculiar languidness, her delicacy and consequent charm? Circus people know how to commercialize the unexpected as is evidenced by the freaks they carry around with them. Beggars, too, when they reveal their disabilities to passers-by, are good psychologists in this respect.

It has happened that the very fact of illness has been the means of discovering a hidden talent. A patient who, while bedridden with a fractured hip, saw grotesque faces and figures in the wall-paper designs of his bedroom, was thereby started on the way toward becoming a sketch artist. In seeking the cause of neurotic disorders, inherent, unsuspected abilities often are brought to light. Such neurotics, naturally, are particularly glad.

Yes, illness and misfortune of all kinds may truly be blessings in disguise to make you glad. One may come face to face with reality for the first time. Suffering, even, may turn out to be a marvelous teacher. It may make us think and think deeply. In searching our souls it can give us the first real insight into life that we have ever had. When we are young and conceited over our vigorous bodies, sound health, ambition and abilities, we tend to lack the seriousness of purpose which a blow from the unexpected usually brings home to us. It may be a cruel awakening; nevertheless, it is an awakening. The unexpected makes us take a sensible view of life. We see where we have made mistakes. It makes us resolve to live differently in the future.

Whenever the unexpected descends upon us the fight-flight mechanism, discussed in Chap. XIV, is brought into play. Small wonder that persons who receive several shocks within a comparatively short space of time use up an unusual amount of reserve energy, which leaves them exhausted or candidates for a case of nerves. If, however, the fight-flight mechanism operates more frequently, but less intensely and deliberately, it becomes a more flexible mechanism because of such operation, while likewise becoming strengthened.

Remember that each time you fight you are behaving in accord with your primitive instincts, which are brave and aggressive in character. Contrariwise, each time you run away you are going counter to the stand that nature has destined you to take in the struggle for existence. Don't forget that the fittest survive and the fittest fight; they don't flee. Therefore, be a fighter; if necessary *look for fight.* In this way you will not only know how to meet the unexpected when it arrives, but you will combat it perfectly and, what is more, automatically. You will have learned how to control your future.

It was that eminent physician, Osler, who said that we are not likely to die of a disease we know we have and which we are watching, but rather of a disease that takes hold unexpectedly because we are not prepared.

Be prepared! Don't think that fate has predestined everything for you; that you were born under an evil or a lucky star; that no matter what you do you can't control your future. If that were true, doctors would be superfluous. Just as you can add ten or more years to your life span by being prepared for the unexpected as regards your health, so you can ward off the often cruel effects of the unexpected upon your feelings and your morale, particularly upon your sensitive neurotic constitution.

Nor should you think you may never be hit by the unexpected because so far you have been spared. Recall what the depression did to thousands. We prepare for death by going to church, selecting a cemetery plot and taking out life insurance. We should, in a similar way, prepare for all possible unforeseen occurrences, good or bad, by being ready as set forth. That is the way to remain glad.

Learn How to Control Your Future

Viscount Morley in his *Recollections* quotes from an essay by John Stuart Mill as follows:

> Next to birth the chief cause of success in life is accident and opportunity. . . . In the situation of most people no degree whatever of good conduct can be counted on for raising them in the world without the aid of fortunate incidents.

But the trouble is most of us get more "bad breaks" than good ones—at least so they seem when unexpectedly they arrive. Although we cannot prevent their occurrence we should suspect that always they may be "just around the corner."

Be ready, therefore, for the future, no matter how much of the unexpected it may carry. It can, and it should be done. You will never regret it!

Chapter XIX

IF IT'S TREATMENT YOU NEED, WHAT KIND?

PREPARE YOURSELF IN THE SAME MANNER when it comes to the matter of treatment. If yours is an established neurosis with symptoms that interfere with your general well-being, not to mention your other relationships in life, *get rid of it!* Individual treatment at the hands of a competent specialist may likewise be desirable if you are merely neurotic, if you have not yet developed an out-and-out neurosis.

Whatever you do, don't just run around from one doctor to another or follow some religious or other cult without seeking basic therapy.

Remember that a neurosis is curable no matter how long you have suffered from it. You must never lose hope. Few neuroses do not respond to the proper kind of treatment fairly soon even though a complete cure may take months. The day is past when a year was no time at all to devote to such a cure. Modern methods and experience in the field of the functional disorders have reduced the treatment period of the average case by two-thirds. Even in the unusually difficult cases—those exceptional ones that prove the rule that all neuroses can be cured—improvement can result.

Bear in mind, too, that by now your neurosis is probably an old friend, although an annoying one, whom you may really be loath to forsake. In other words, your neurotic symptoms have been a kind of prop for you for years. They have often come in handy as an excuse for your failure to obtain or hold a job, to get yourself married, actually to knuckle down to business, whatever the issue.

A neurosis can be a wonderful alibi. It's a backlog to which you can retreat and behind which you can hide. It draws attention to yourself and creates interest, even sympathy. And if you think your own particular neurosis is the most extraordinary and baffling one ever encountered by medical science—which is not an uncommon opinion and is never true—it actually can boost your ego.

Being convinced, however, that you can't forget your neurosis or that you cannot dispel it through distraction, change of job, a new family setup or the power of the will, what kind of treatment should you seek?

The First World War helped to put the recognition of mental maladjustments on the map; the Second World War has definitely made people psychiatric-minded. The publicity that the neuroses and their treatment has received in newspapers and magazines is enormous. In the main, this is excellent, but it also has had its drawbacks. People are becoming acquainted with so many kinds of treatment these days that they scarcely know which way to turn.

There is *hypnotism,* for example. One hears it mentioned as though it were a brand-new method. Yet Sigmund Freud himself, founder of the psychoanalytic school, used hypnosis in the early days and discarded it.

First of all, not everyone can be hypnotized. Secondly, such controlled suggestion changes nothing that is basic regarding the causes of a neurosis. These causes are laid down over the years from childhood on up in a cumulative way. The symptoms of neurosis are merely indicative signs, "symbols," as the psychiatrists say, of these causes which are always maladjustments in the emotional sphere due to the child's individualized reaction to his environment. No form of treatment that does not *resurrect* buried and forgotten memories in the unconscious mind, make them conscious in order to take the guilt out of them, then integrates the new personality that develops, can cure a neurosis.

Hypnosis merely imposes the will of the hypnotist upon his subject, adds more material—even if it be constructive—to the unconscious and does not change in any appreciable way the immature, unfinished business to be found there. You cannot run away from yourself. Although hypnosis often is helpful in children too young to understand psychoanalysis, it produces no permanent curative effects in neurotic adults.

I, myself, employed hypnotism when I first specialized in psychiatry. Then, when psychoanalysis appeared upon the horizon, many psychiatrists, myself included, passed through a phase where we used both hypnosis and psychoanalysis in a particular case, hoping through hypnosis to reach deeply repressed memories and to break down strong resistances to cure or change that the patient might present. But the combination did not work satisfactorily.

After all, to undergo effective treatment for a neurosis is like experiencing a reeducation. No man or woman thinks and feels the same after he has been analyzed simply because he has at last got rid of his emotional immaturity of which he probably was himself unaware. Indeed, those who have carried along a neurosis all their lives, as they would drag a ball and chain, can't imagine what it means to be free of it. They have not as yet lived at all. Once they do the sheer joy of living is unmistakable. Then they are glad!

Army hospitals have been trying various means of giving quick aid to men suffering from so-called "battle fatigue." In the First World War the term used was "shell shock." These reactions of loss of memory, guilt, confusion, weakness, fear or panic, etc., are neurotic in character.

The use of sodium pentothal and other drugs to induce a state of partial or complete narcosis, during which violently repressed memories, conflicts and other emotions are allowed to drain off, is meeting with success. Even in these cases, however, some form of psychoanalysis is employed to reeducate the personality and to prevent, if possible, the danger of recurrence. This combination technique, so to speak, is known as "narcosynthesis."

Which brings to mind "shock therapy" so often mentioned in connection with mind disturbances.

A drug called metrazol was first employed in this connection, injections producing a convulsive seizure of short duration. Insulin also has been administered in a similar way and with similar results. Electric shock has since grown more popular. In the last-named a weak electric current is passed through the patient's brain by means of electrodes placed at the temples. The treatment is almost instantaneous and the patient suffers no pain. Unconsciousness occurs, followed by a convulsive seizure of short duration. Sometimes curare is used to diminish the convulsion. The patient usually recovers consciousness in ten to twenty minutes and does not recollect anything that has happened to him. So-called "ambulatory shock" is also being used. Here the current is weaker still and the patient may not require hospitalization.

That shock therapy, irrespective of its kind and the frequency of its use, has opened up an entirely new field in the treatment of the psychoses there can be no question. Personally, I do not recommend it as routine treatment for the neuroses. It can be helpful in certain cases, the differentiation of which does not properly belong here. In fact, shock treatment does not always produce improvement or cure even in *psychotic* individuals. More research along these lines is being pursued. The wisdom of its application should be left entirely to the judgment of the psychiatrist in charge. At any rate, a certain amount of analytic probing should be used in addition.

Psychoanalysis still remains the means, par excellence, for the treatment of neurotic states and the neuroses. This form of therapy has spread throughout the world, and its literature of thousands of books and many more thousands of articles is steadily mounting. Every large medical center has its psychoanalysts or psychiatrists who employ psychoanalysis as a form of treatment. Freudian analysis is still universally practiced, although the modifications of Jung, Adler and others are employed. Psychiatrists—these men, by the way, are always M.D.'s—have a way of using analysis according to their own individual concepts. After all, the practice of psychiatry is an art rather than an exact science.

The chief difficulty encountered in treating all patients with psychoanalysis is "resistance." By this is meant the fight which the patient puts up—usually he is not aware of what he is doing—against changing the habit patterns of his inner nature.

To be sure, he wants to be rid of his handicapping symptoms, but on his own terms. He is not always willing to change his point of view on life completely enough. Furthermore, when repressions, which originally were painful experiences, are brought to conscious recognition, he may feel that he is getting worse and may even wish to discontinue treatment entirely. Or the patient may suddenly declare that he is sure his is an incurable case because it is of such long standing or because he has come to the conclusion that his condition is hereditary or because he has learned that insanity appears in his family tree. All alibis, of course, and nonsense to boot!

To be sure, reactions such as these, if they occur, are only temporary in nature. The handling of such resistances are, nevertheless, the psychiatrist's most difficult task.

The question often asked by a patient about to be analyzed is: "Suppose we do find repressions, complexes, conflicts and whatnot in my unconscious mind, doctor, and we bring them to the surface, to conscious recognition—how will that cure me?" Which is fair enough. It is hoped that the following case will make this clear.

A man of twenty-nine was suffering from severe self-consciousness. Ever since he could remember he had shunned social gatherings, girls, restaurants and all public places. From work he went home to his room where he read and listened to the radio. It was a monotonous existence if ever there was one.

In the course of analysis he was able to remember—all this had been blotted out for years—that when he was twelve years old he had a teacher for whom he developed a typical adolescent "crush." Although his mother was a stern and undemonstrative woman who never gave the child any affection, this teacher was warm and motherly. He used to think how much he would have liked to have *her* for a mother. At night, while in bed, the boy would phantasize about this teacher. He would wonder how it would be if she were lying next to him, holding him in her arms.

All would probably have been well had not *guilt* entered his mind. Having heard about sex from other boys, also feeling guilty about knowing such things, he began to think that he was entertaining sex thoughts about his teacher that were wrong.

Then one day the teacher called upon him in class to recite. Although a bright pupil who always did his homework and knew his lessons, he found himself confused and blushing. He kept thinking of what teacher would think of him if she knew his secret thoughts and wishes. He could not say a word. The teacher, surprised, told him to sit down. From that moment his self-consciousness started.

The point is that the patient had totally forgotten both the incident mentioned and his adoration for his teacher. It was entirely repressed. Nevertheless, this unconscious guilt was still influencing him, making him feel that he was different although he did not know why.

When this complex, this emotionally mixed-up state, was finally resolved and made simple and understandable, I asked the patient if he still thought he was in love with this teacher of years gone by and if he still thought he would like to have her in bed holding him in her arms.

He laughed. "Say, doc," he said, "don't you think I would now prefer a younger woman?"

In other words, in the light of his adult intelligence and experience, what was so vital to him as a child ceased to be important as a mature man. And that's the way, in a general sense, that people who are psychoanalyzed are cured.

A single, dramatic incident such as I have outlined is not always the root or main cause of a neurosis. Even the patient in question had other maladjustments in childhood that needed attention. The man really suffered from a mother fixation. A point of view of life, religious upsets—almost any intangible emotional reaction—may constitute the cause or causes of a neurosis.

The criticism is often voiced that psychoanalysis deals too much with sex. Is it not true, however, that more guilt, misinformation and incompatibility regarding sex exists than about anything else? Don't assail analysis for being compelled to stress sex—in fact, it only does so when necessary. Criticize nature or the social set up in which we live.

Thorough treatment of neurotic conditions of all kinds frequently includes attention to blood pressure, vitamin deficiency (especially B_1), diet in general, exercise, entertainment and social contacts, to revitalizing the nerve cells themselves and to other strictly organic complaints in addition to attention directed to the mind, as such, alone. Each case varies.

What happens if you keep your neurosis, try to overcome it with will power and "sweat it out"? Well, you won't go insane, that's certain. You will, however, court the possibility of your symptoms growing worse. What's more, even if you overcome some symptoms, new ones may be added. And, of course, if the progress of the neurosis is not checked, a nervous breakdown possibly may result. When this happens the patient is so upset and exhausted that he no longer is able to function adequately, and he must be put to bed and treated as one would any sick, incapacitated person.

Therefore, if it's treatment you need, be sure to get it! But see to it that you obtain the correct kind, the kind that is individualized, that does not merely stress one part of you but that considers your mind and all the other organs of the body as a single unit, a whole.

Chapter XX

CONSIDER OVERCOMPENSATION AND CHEER UP

HAVE YOU EVER STOOD BESIDE A STREAM, wondering if you could jump across it, in fact, feeling that you couldn't? The chances are that all of a sudden something within you urged you to try and, not only were you able to jump the water safely, you actually jumped farther than was necessary.

That is *overcompensation.*

Have you ever been fearful of meeting someone—perhaps a social celebrity or an employer—only to find that, once you got started, you succeeded in handling the situation beyond your fondest expectations?

That, too, is *overcompensation.*

Now consider a handicap more serious than temporary physical timidity or mental embarrassment. Suppose you are suffering from inferiority convictions to such an extent that they thwart your ambition, undermine your efficiency, interfere with the gratification of your love life and, all in all, render you generally miserable.

What would you say if someone told you that the traits that hold you back can be turned into traits that hurtle you into success? That not only can you *rid* yourself of your handicaps but that, in addition, each separate devastating inferiority conviction actually can be changed into a definite and pronounced superiority?

A paradox, you say, almost impossible to believe? Not when you study the psychology underlying overcompensation. Indeed, due to this astounding dynamic force many, if not most, of the world's greatest achievements have been effected. It is overcompensation that can make every neurotic both successful and glad.

Consider the case of Clifford W. Beers. He was insane, confined in an asylum. Did he, after release, consider himself hopelessly handicapped? Not by a long shot! He wrote a book, since made famous, called *A Mind That Found Itself*, and it sold by the thousands. Still not satisfied, still overcompensating, he went ahead and founded the National Committee for Mental Hygiene. It is no exaggeration to state that were it not for this organization, and specifically through the personal and tireless efforts of Beers, humane and scientific treatment of the insane would not be what it is today. Take Dr. Trudeau. Not only did he cure his own handicap of tuberculosis by braving the winter cold of the Adirondacks, he went ahead and established there what later became a world-famous sanatorium, thereby proving, once and for all, the value of fresh air in checking this hitherto baffling disease. Then there was Joseph Conrad. Up to the age of twenty he could not write a word of English because he was born and raised in Poland. His determination was so strong, however, that his overcompensation finally made him one of the greatest novelists and stylists in the language. Sometimes he would write and rewrite for hours until he had mastered what he considered a few satisfactory sentences. Lastly, note how Disraeli overcompensated. He was a Jew and despised. But before he got through with the world he had become Prime Minister of England, with everybody showing him respect, his former enemies in particular acknowledging his superiority.

Perhaps you recall the story of Javert in Victor Hugo's *Les Misérables.* The author, with profound psychological insight, has this character explain why he became a police inspector, and a stern and cruel one at that. His father had been a criminal, a hunted man; the son resolved to become a pursuer instead of one pursued. Again overcompensation!

How much the above nonfiction personalities were motivated automatically and unconsciously, I am not prepared to say. For it is true that the mind often does the job of overcompensation for us when little or no conscious effort is in evidence.

When the will is exercised, however, the result is even more striking. Consciousness, being the intermediary between the unconscious and the outside world, can exert a directing influence toward practical ends in a more telling way. In other words, whereas unconscious, automatic overcompensation may prove successful, it nevertheless is more or less of a haphazard process, and hence may fail.

Imagine, therefore, what actually *you can accomplish for yourself.* The thought itself should make you glad.

On the other hand, you must do more than phantasize. You must get down to business and *do something!* Frankly, it is up to you to take your handicaps in hand. It is your duty to try to conquer them. Every handicap you possess should be looked upon as a direct and personal *challenge.* The more neurotic you are, the more symptoms you possess, the greater that challenge!

When you stood by the stream wondering whether you could jump across, you were being challenged. When you were afraid to meet someone a voice from within nevertheless dared you to try. Nature, you see, wants you to express yourself fully, wholly; to contact reality and harmonize with it 100 per cent. You really have everything in your favor when you set out to compensate because you are *assisting* nature.

Small wonder, once the brakes on expression are released, that the energy so long pent up—so powerful simply because it has been confined—rushes you forward and up to heights you scarcely dreamed you ever would reach. Small wonder that when neurotics achieve, they achieve signally.

Neglect is one of the major causes of all handicaps; neglect in developing an inherent ability that has been lagging behind.

If, for instance, you are convinced you cannot swim or make a speech, obviously what you should have done is take swimming or elocution lessons. You should never have neglected such essentials. Actually receive such special training, however, and the interest plus the satisfaction thus created will probably impel you to wish to excel. Two illustrations of this come to mind. In the one, the man afterward entered a long-distance swimming race, while in the other the woman became a teacher of dramatics.

Although we should blame ourselves for not trying to turn a recognized handicap into an asset, we often are not to blame that we possess such a handicap. Often the need for developing a certain side of our personality was not apparent to those who trained and educated us.

A girl of wealthy parents may never take an interest in cooking or sewing because her mother does not encourage it; the mother believes that her daughter will always employ servants. Yet such a girl may fall in love with a poor man and find herself handicapped. If a boy is brought up on a farm and his parents intend him to be a farmer, they may not attempt to develop the social side of his character. Such a boy conceivably may grow up diffident and shy.

In addition to neglect, a frequent cause for handicaps is a *psychic trauma.* By this is meant a mental or emotional hurt, or both, which acts as a shock to the nervous system, produces an indelible impression and influences the individual throughout his life.

Two general types of such traumata are to be recognized. One is a sudden and unexpected shock, such as overwhelmingly bad news; the other a series of lesser traumata experienced over a long period.

A patient was continually scolded by her mother for being awkward with her hands; still another for indifference about her personal appearance. The first girl deliberately took courses in modeling and painting in order to exercise and train the small muscle groups of the hand and in the end became a sculptress; the second afterward blossomed forth as a dress designer.

Ask the average person suffering with a handicap to think back to childhood for the cause and he probably will answer: "I have tried that and failed." Or he may say: "It seems to me I have had it all my life." But keep nagging him and before long he actually finds the cause or he recalls incidents that lead up to it.

An excellent method is to write down what might be called the "purple patches" (pleasurable or otherwise) of your life—that is, incidents in childhood that impressed you, that had a telling effect. It may be disappointment in a love affair, an exceptionally low mark at school, regret over some youthful indiscretion, misplaced confidence in a friend, loss of money or a job, inability to achieve an ambition. Any one of these, and many others besides, may turn out to be the starting point for discovering the real cause of your difficulty. Indeed, often it is the earliest memories you can resurrect that give a clue.

Giving way to a handicap is really surrendering to an infantile fixation. As you know, this means that despite your adult years you are still acting emotionally like a child. It is a basic neurotic trait. Think of that and it will help.

Remember also that you are what you are today because of everything you have been from the cradle up to the present moment. Life is a continuous process. In fashioning that continuum, in shaping its course, in setting the milestones of success as well as failure, no incident should be adjudged, from the psychological standpoint, as trivial or inconsequential.

A man of forty was pronouncedly lacking in self-confidence. He possessed energy, ambition and originality, but he would always be stopped in his tracks by the devastating thought: "If I do that, what will people think?" In seeking the cause, by letting his mind drift into the past, he recalled that he was brought up in a small town and that his grandmother, with whom he lived, was forever coercing him and warning him to consider the neighbors. "But I live in a large city now," he finally concluded, "even the people who live on the same floor with me in my apartment don't care a rap what I think, say or do. I'll be hanged if I let myself still be influenced by the narrow-minded ideas of my grandmother. I am acting as I did when a child." That was enough to eradicate the handicap.

One might think that the longer a handicap is in existence the more difficult it is to overcompensate. As a matter of fact, a long-standing defect, neurotic or otherwise, may in the end result in greater overcompensation for the very reason that in trying to overcome it more momentum is developed.

Nor should you think that only a few selected handicaps can be corrected and changed from liabilities into assets. Some variety of overcompensation, either directly of an opposite nature, or indirectly of a less direct compensatory nature but still making for success, can be found.

Of the latter, Lafcadio Hearn is an illuminating example. He was a sickly man, blind in one eye, in constant dread that he also would lose the sight of the other. His health could not be improved nor his eyesight. In short, he was incurable. He claimed, however, that his unusual type of mind was the result of his illness. "The owner of pure horse flesh," he declared, "never purchased the power of discerning half-lights. In its separation of the spiritual from the physical portion of existence, severe sickness is often invaluable in the revelation it bestows of the undercurrents of existence." Knowing this and reading Hearn, no one could doubt but that his work, so discerning and sensitive, represents overcompensation.[1]

Various types of inferiority, self-consciousness, oversensitiveness, timidity, fear of the future, doubt, worry about making

[1] For additional examples of overcompensation in illness, consult Chap. XVIII.

good in marriage, physical weakness and cowardice, are among the common handicaps encountered. When overcompensated, however, the inferior may become bold salesmen, the self-conscious actors, the oversensitive book agents, the timid lawyers, those with an unwarranted fear of the future may retire from business at fifty; the "doubting Thomases" may become leaders in some new movement; those afraid of marriage may become the finest wives and mothers; the physically weak may develop muscles like a Sandow; and the cowardly may become soldiers and policemen. Nor do they always realize what they have accomplished or that they are neurotic.

The above overcompensations may not be the ones you, yourself, would choose. Nor would you, should you be a woman, care to change from a "wallflower" into a coquette (an actual case, by the way). But there are so many ways of accomplishing something desirable via overcompensation that with a little study of individual desires and needs a solution can always be found. What's more, if you realize the neurotic element in your handicap, hence its cause, the overcompensatory adjustment is so much easier and more effective.

As a rule one feels that it is more difficult to overcompensate for a physical handicap than for a mental or emotional one. On the whole, this is true. Yet see what Helen Keller has done with her blindness. Consider, too, that Theodore Roosevelt, the elder, was a delicate boy. He was sent to a ranch out West. Through overcompensation he became the symbol of the "big stick." Paderewski, surprisingly enough, had weak fingers. Overcompensation made of him one of the world's greatest pianists.

Even poverty is surmountable. Think how Spinoza, Rousseau, Goldsmith and Dr. Johnson struggled against it and won. Remember, too, the financial losses that Sir Walter Scott and our own Mark Twain suffered. But they did not give up. In fact, poverty often has been the incentive for superior accomplishment. It is said that Mascagni wrote no music so fine as *Cavalleria Rusticana,* done while he was poor. And is it not true that some of the biggest fortunes of the present day have been built up by poor boys? Is this not overcompensation?

It is interesting to note, too, how frequently overcompensation reveals itself in an artist's work. Consider Eugene O'Neill's plays. By nature he is shy and retiring but his dramas are the essence of strength. To look at one of MacMonnies' statues, such as his "Civic Virtue" or his Marne memorial, one might picture him as a six-footer, built like a wrestler. Actually, however, he looks quite different. In fact, the greatest works of art often do not reflect the nature of their author photographically, but in an overcompensatory way for some deficiency, handicap or weakness.

It must be remembered that no person ever developed to capacity, not even as regards the specialized work he is doing. Besides, millions of brain cells—on the right side of the cerebrum, especially—remain dormant throughout life for want of use. Theoretically, we can do about what we wish with our minds.

To overcome a handicap and overcompensate is much the same as consciously and deliberately setting out to overcome a superstition. We will say that you are afraid to pass under a ladder. But suppose you defy the superstition and do it anyway? You may feel uneasy for a few hours or a few days. To your surprise, perhaps, nothing dreadful happens to you.

This gives you courage. You try the ladder stunt again. Still you find yourself unharmed. After a while you look for ladders; you delight in walking under them; your ego has been pepped up and you defy all the demons that may be! *Courage begets courage in the same way that fear begets fear.* Each time you succeed you automatically become bolder to try again.

Put your *will* to work; don't falter and you *can't* fail! All you have to do is keep at it long enough. What happens inside your unconscious mind is this: First you neutralize, then obliterate, old reflex arcs—in other words, habits that have throttled you and prevented you from being what you want to be. Next new reflex arcs come into being to replace the old ones, new ones designed to make you efficient, that will carry you where you want to go, that will make you glad.

Suppose a person is suggestible, too much so for his own good. Let us assume that whatever he reads in the editorial columns of a newspaper influences and sways him. Should he read two papers with divergent opinions the same day, he is in a muddle. We may say in this case that the reflex arcs regarding response to external stimuli have deteriorated him to a mere "yes-man." His reflexes have made him agree before he thinks; after a while he no longer is able to think, at least for himself. That is the sort of handicap that needs a stiff dose of overcompensation.

What can such a person do? Deliberately argue every point made in every editorial read, either with someone else or with himself. New reflex arcs will soon be established—in fact, with surprising speed—and the spell of suggestibility broken.

I know a man like that. It all started with a country schoolteacher who, to meet every argument of his class and make it easy for himself, would declare: "Look it up in the book. If it is printed, it is true!"

This man followed the recipe given above and it worked like a charm. Now he is a judge on the bench and so definitely resistive is he to suggestion that he seldom makes an important decision without "sleeping over it," without weighing and considering most carefully every argument pro and con, and until he has made up his own mind to his own satisfaction.

You probably have heard that when an aviator has a crack-up he goes up into the air again about as quickly as he can. He says he doesn't want the accident to "get him." The psychiatrist says the aviator does not want reflex arcs to be established which will keep him afraid.

One of our best known magazine editors told me how terribly shy he was when a boy, so much so that he used to be teased about it and when he was introduced to other boys he blushed. "But I made up my mind that when I grew up I'd know more people than anybody else. Well, maybe I haven't exactly made good on that boast, yet I do know a whale of a lot of authors—and enjoy it—and that's one good reason why I hold my job." This gentleman's destructive reflex arcs that carried fear surely gave way to constructive ones that now yield pleasure as well as profit.

Overcompensation often occurs automatically in an emergency. When the steamship *Dixie* was in distress on a coral reef, the water as high as the cabin bunks and baggage floating around in all directions, this is what one of the passengers afterward said happened: "We all were of the opinion that we would finally be carried down. But there was no hysteria. We all sang!"

Overcompensation may also benefit others as well as the individual himself. I once remarked to a former patient that he paid his bills with astonishing speed. "That's because my father was in debt all his life," he replied. "To this day I shudder when I think of the stream of bill collectors that used to ring the front doorbell and whom I had to put off continually with one excuse or another."

There is often a humorous side to overcompensation when you realize that its motivation is likely to be of an opposite nature. It may then be properly termed a *defense mechanism.* A person may boast about how hard he works when, deep down, the cause is laziness. Likewise, marked tidiness and cleanliness may signify overcompensation for disorderliness and uncleanliness; excessive politeness an overcompensation for rudeness; a pleasant manner for bad temper; talkativeness for a fundamental dislike of people; self-discipline for carelessness; thriftiness for a spendthrift nature; kindness for cruelty; generosity for avariciousness.

Lastly, overcompensation may carry danger, likewise of the defense variety. Fast automobile driving, beyond the limits of safety, undoubtedly denotes a weak ego. By passing everybody else on the road, by tooting the horn loud and often, the driver's ego is boosted. Dictators, particularly the harsh and cruel ones, are motivated by a similar personal psychology. Inferiority, strange as it may seem, may overcompensate into unbridled pride, audacity and self-assurance. And sometimes it goes too far. Then the dictator is no more.

In fact, since overcompensation is really a *marked* and

excessive compensation, always suspect exaggerated behavior of any kind as having been brought about, consciously or unconsciously, by a quite different, an opposite, form of behavior.

No person is well developed in all his intellectual faculties or in all the components of his emotional make-up. Particularly is this true of neurotics. One person is, relatively speaking, poor in drawing logical conclusions or his imagination is not readily aroused. Or, in the emotional sphere, his feelings are easily hurt or he becomes embarrassed without justification. In other words, we all have handicaps to greater or less degree. These, too, can be overcome—and in the same way as the more pronounced varieties—through the principle of overcompensation.

An attempt should invariably be made to bring weak abilities up to the level of our best ones. This makes for valuable balancing factors and enriches and rounds out our lives. That is why I repeat that every handicap should be considered by you as a challenge. Your real, true, inner, unconscious self wants so earnestly to make you do something about it. And, just as in a family the sickly child, although perhaps at first not welcomed, afterward gets most of the love and attention and becomes the favorite child, so you, as the head of your own mental household, should pay particular and solicitous attention to *your* handicap. Don't be afraid or ashamed of it. Look upon it as a cry for help. Respect your handicap, give it the required attention until it becomes your truly favorite trait instead of the one you have always wanted to hide.

Nor am I talking mere inspiration psychology. I am not trying to give you a "pep talk." The mind is a machine. Your various group thoughts and feelings are integral components of that machine. Your automobile does not run smoothly if the air and gas are not properly mixed in the carburetor. There is choking and sputtering, the car jolts and halts, there may be explosions.

The situation is identical when one of your component mental parts is out of harmony with the rest. It wants so much to be heard. It wishes to express itself. It wants to be given a chance. That is why it makes such a fuss; why your handicap produces fears, discouragement and panic. *That is why you are neurotic!* A devastating emotion is tagged onto the handicap in order that you may constantly and effectively be reminded to get busy.

That is why, also, once you do pay attention, everything is in your favor for success; that you quite naturally and easily overcompensate; that you excel where once you felt dismayed.

The start in overcompensation, as in everything else, is the hardest. Persevere, however; don't give up. Grapple with your handicaps, whatever their nature; conquer them. The energy thus released does the rest.

Overcompensation has made the weak strong; the inefficient efficient; the inferior superior; the fearsome bold; the sickly healthy; the despairing hopeful. In other words, it has made the neurotic glad!

A chain is as strong as its weakest link. Repair that link, weld it, and that particular link becomes stronger than any of the others. That is overcompensation!

The more neurotic you are the better adjusted you can become. Every devastating symptom you possess can be changed into an outstanding asset of opposite character.

Consider Overcompensation and Cheer Up

You should be glad that you possess so many factors that can be turned to your advantage. At least something is brewing inside of you. Your mind is neither static nor dead. You are in a state of flux; in a condition of change. You won't remain the way you are because you can't. You will become a being who will laugh heartily when, later on, he looks back and compares what he is then with what he was.

That, too, will be overcompensation!

Chapter XXI

THEN FOLLOW THESE FIVE SIMPLE RULES—THAT'S ALL!

IN CONCLUDING THIS VOLUME—WHICH SHOULD prove not merely an inspiration to you but a definite and practical handbook as well—permit me to quote from the keynote address made by Dr. Joseph V. Collins, one of the founders of the Neurological Institute, on the occasion of its twenty-fifth anniversary:

> Submit to being called a neurotic [he declared] for then you belong to that splendid and pitiable family which is the salt of the earth. All the greatest things we know have come to us from neurotics. It is they, and they only, who have founded religions and created works of art. . . .
>
> It is the psychoneurotics who have painted the pictures that have lasted from the time of El Greco. Just as sure as the Mississippi River flows from Lake Itasca, all modern art flows from El Greco. Just as sure as Leonardo da Vinci existed, all modern applications of physics stem from him.
>
> You can't name a poet, whether it be Whitman or Poe in this country, or Stephen Collins Foster or Swinburne, but that you find a psychoneurotic. . . .
>
> Never will the world be conscious of how much it owes to the neurotics, nor above all what they have suffered in order to bestow its gifts on it. We enjoy fine music, beautiful pictures, a thousand exquisite things, but we do not know what it cost those who wrought them in sleeplessness, tears, spasmodic laughter, asthma, epilepsy, terror of death and worse than these.

Then Follow These Five Simple Rules—That's All!

But the time is past when you must suffer as did the great, and the neurotic generally, of days gone by. The science of psychiatry is only, comparatively speaking, a recent branch of learning.

Frankly, if you are neurotic and you continue to suffer, you have only yourself to blame. If you are neurotic you can help yourself. If you are laboring under the weight of a full-fledged and severe neurosis specialists are at hand.

In any case, *follow these five simple rules.* Remind yourself of them morning and night. If necessary, paste them inside your hat!

ANALYZE YOURSELF

STOP FEELING GUILTY

GIVE YOUR EGO A BOOST

TURN YOUR HANDICAPS INTO ASSETS

PROFIT BY YOUR NEUROSIS

Then

BE GLAD!